ORTHOPEDIC CLINICS OF NORTH AMERICA

www.orthopedic.theclinics.com

Arthritis and Related Conditions

October 2019 • Volume 50 • Number 4

ELSEVIER

1600 John F. Kennedy Boulevard • Suite 1800 • Philadelphia, Pennsylvania, 19103-2899.

http://www.orthopedic.theclinics.com

ORTHOPEDIC CLINICS OF NORTH AMERICA Volume 50, Number 4
October 2019 ISSN 0030-5898, ISBN-13: 978-0-323-71040-4

Editor: Lauren Boyle
Developmental Editor: Kristen Helm

Orthopedic Clinics of North America (ISSN 0030-5898) is published quarterly by Elsevier Inc., 360 Park Avenue South, New York, NY 10010-1710. Months of issue are January, April, July, and October. Business and Editorial Offices: 1600 John F. Kennedy Blvd., Suite 1800, Philadelphia, PA 19103-2899. Customer Service Office: 3251 Riverport Lane, Maryland Heights, MO 63043. Periodicals postage paid at New York, NY and additional mailing offices. Subscription prices are $341.00 per year for (US individuals), $749.00 per year for (US institutions), $403.00 per year (Canadian individuals), $914.00 per year (Canadian institutions), $466.00 per year (international individuals), $914.00 per year (international institutions), $100.00 per year (US students), $220.00 per year (Canadian and international students). Foreign air speed delivery is included in all *Clinics* subscription prices. All prices are subject to change without notice. **POSTMASTER:** Send change of address to *Orthopedic Clinics of North America*, **Elsevier Health Sciences Division, Subscription Customer Service, 3251 Riverport Lane, Maryland Heights, MO 63043. Customer Service (orders, claims, online, change of address): Elsevier Health Sciences Division, Subscription Customer Service, 3251 Riverport Lane, Maryland Heights, MO 63043. Tel: 1-800-654-2452 (U.S. and Canada); 314-447-8871 (outside U.S. and Canada). Fax: 314-447-8029. E-mail:** journalscustomerservice-usa@elsevier.com **(for print support);** journalsonlinesupport-usa@elsevier.com **(for online support).**

Reprints. For copies of 100 or more, of articles in this publication, please contact the Commercial Reprints Department, Elsevier Inc., 360 Park Avenue South, New York, NY 10010-1710. Tel.: 212-633-3874; Fax: 212-633-3820; E-mail: reprints@elsevier.com.

Orthopedic Clinics of North America is covered in *MEDLINE/PubMed (Index Medicus)*, Cinahl, Excerpta Medica, and Cumulative Index to Nursing and Allied Health Literature.

EDITORIAL BOARD

CONTRIBUTORS

AUTHORS

SAMUEL B. ADAMS, MD
Associate Residency Program Director,
Co-Chief, Division of Foot and Ankle
Surgery, Director of Foot and Ankle
Research, Assistant Professor, Department
of Orthopaedic Surgery, Duke University
Medical Center, Durham, North Carolina,
USA

JOSE CARLOS ALCERRO, MD
Orthopedic Surgery, Adult Joint
Reconstruction, Instituto Hondureño
de Seguridad Social, Tegucigalpa,
Honduras

ALEXANDER W. ALEEM, MD
Assistant Professor, Shoulder and Elbow
Surgery, Department of Orthopaedic
Surgery, Washington University School of
Medicine, St Louis, Missouri, USA

HUSAM AL-RUMAIH, MD, MPH
Foot and Ankle Fellow, Department of
Orthopaedics, University of British Columbia,
Footbridge Centre for Integrated
Orthopaedic Care, Vancouver, British
Columbia, Canada

VINCENT ATHAS, BS
Texas Tech University School of Medicine,
Texas Tech University Health Science Center,
Lubbock, Texas, USA

SCOT N. BAUMAN, PT, DPT
Shelbourne Knee Center at Community East
Hospital, Indianapolis, Indiana, USA

RODNEY W. BENNER, MD
Shelbourne Knee Center at Community East
Hospital, Indianapolis, Indiana, USA

KAREN M. BOVID, MD
Assistant Professor, Department
of Orthopaedic Surgery, Western
Michigan University Homer Stryker M.D.
School of Medicine, Kalamazoo, Michigan,
USA

TYLER J. BROLIN, MD
Clinical Instructor, Department of
Orthopaedic Surgery, The University
of Tennessee Health Science Center,
Campbell Clinic, Memphis, Tennessee,
USA

DANIEL W. BROWN, MD
Department of Orthopaedic Surgery and
Biomedical Engineering, Le Bonheur
Children's Hospital, The University of
Tennessee Health Science Center,
Campbell Clinic, Memphis, Tennessee,
USA

JAMES H. CALANDRUCCIO, MD
Associate Professor, Department of
Orthopaedic Surgery and Biomedical
Engineering, The University of Tennessee
Health Science Center, Campbell Clinic,
Memphis, Tennessee, USA

DAVID C. CARVER, MD
Fellow, Lake Tahoe Sports Medicine
Fellowship, Zephyr Cove, Nevada,
USA

JACOB T. DAVIS, MD
Orthopaedic Trauma Fellow, Department
of Orthopaedic Surgery and Biomedical
Engineering, The University of Tennessee
Health Science Center, Campbell Clinic,
Regional One Health Hospital, The
Campbell Foundation, Memphis, Tennessee,
USA

TINKER GRAY, MA
Shelbourne Knee Center at Community
East Hospital, Indianapolis, Indiana,
USA

PETER R. HENNING, MD
Orthopaedic Resident, Department of
Orthopaedic Surgery and Biomedical
Engineering, The University of Tennessee
Health Science Center, Campbell Clinic,
Memphis, Tennessee, USA

LUCKSHMANA JEYASEELAN, MBBS, BSc, FRCS(Tr&Orth)
Foot and Ankle Fellow, Department of Orthopaedics, University of British Columbia, Footbridge Centre for Integrated Orthopaedic Care, Vancouver, British Columbia, Canada

LAWAL A. LABARAN, BS
University of Illinois College of Medicine, Chicago, Illinois, USA

CARLOS JESUS LAVERNIA, MD
Orthopedic Surgery, Adult Joint Reconstruction, Arthritis Surgery Research Foundation, Coral Gables, Florida, USA

SIDDHANT K. MEHTA, MD, PhD
Clinical Fellow, Shoulder and Elbow Surgery, Department of Orthopaedic Surgery, Washington University School of Medicine, St Louis, Missouri, USA

MARY D. MOORE, MD
Associate Professor, Department of Pediatrics, Central Michigan University College of Medicine, Mount Pleasant, Michigan, USA

ADAM NORRIS
Shelbourne Knee Center at Community East Hospital, Indianapolis, Indiana, USA

EUGENE C. NWANKWO Jr, MS
Department of Orthopedic Surgery, Duke University Medical Center, Durham, North Carolina, USA; Texas Tech University School of Medicine, Texas Tech University Health Science Center, Lubbock, Texas, USA

STEVE OLSON, MD
Department of Orthopedic Surgery, Duke University Medical Center, Durham, North Carolina, USA

MURRAY J. PENNER, MD, FRCSC
Clinical Professor, Department of Orthopaedics, University of British Columbia, Footbridge Centre for Integrated Orthopaedic Care, Vancouver, British Columbia, Canada

HUAI MING PHEN, MBBS
Orthopaedic Surgery Resident, Emory University School of Medicine, Grady Memorial Hospital, Atlanta, Georgia, USA

MARTIN W. ROCHE, MD
Holy Cross Hospital, Orthopedic Research Institute, Fort Lauderdale, Florida, USA

MATTHEW I. RUDLOFF, MD
Assistant Professor, Department of Orthopaedic Surgery and Biomedical Engineering, The University of Tennessee Health Science Center, Campbell Clinic, Regional One Health Hospital, The Campbell Foundation, Memphis, Tennessee, USA

MARA L. SCHENKER, MD
Assistant Professor of Orthopaedic Surgery, Director of Orthopaedic Trauma Research, Emory Orthopaedic Trauma and Fracture, Emory University School of Medicine, Grady Memorial Hospital, Atlanta, Georgia, USA

BENJAMIN W. SHEFFER, MD
Instructor, Department of Orthopaedic Surgery and Biomedical Engineering, Le Bonheur Children's Hospital, The University of Tennessee Health Science Center, Campbell Clinic, Memphis, Tennessee, USA

K. DONALD SHELBOURNE, MD
Shelbourne Knee Center at Community East Hospital, Indianapolis, Indiana, USA

SAM SI-HYEONG PARK, MD, MASc, FRCSC
Foot and Ankle Fellow, Department of Orthopaedics, University of British Columbia, Footbridge Centre for Integrated Orthopaedic Care, Vancouver, British Columbia, Canada

COLIN W. SWIGLER, MD
Orthopaedic Resident, Department of Orthopaedic Surgery and Biomedical Engineering, The University of Tennessee Health Science Center, Campbell Clinic, Memphis, Tennessee, USA

RUSHABH M. VAKHARIA, MD
Holy Cross Hospital, Orthopedic Research Institute, Fort Lauderdale, Florida, USA

ANDREA VELJKOVIC, MD, MPH, FRCSC
Associate Clinical Professor, Department of Orthopaedics, University of British Columbia, Footbridge Centre for Integrated Orthopaedic Care, Vancouver, British Columbia, Canada

WILLIAM JACOB WELLER, MD
Instructor, Department of Orthopaedic
Surgery and Biomedical Engineering, The
University of Tennessee Health Science
Center, Campbell Clinic, Memphis,
Tennessee, USA

KEVIN J. WING, MD, FRCSC
Clinical Professor, Department of
Orthopaedics, University of British Columbia,
Footbridge Centre for Integrated
Orthopaedic Care, Vancouver, British
Columbia, Canada

JOHN C. WU, MD
Hand Fellow, Department of Orthopaedic
Surgery and Biomedical Engineering, The
University of Tennessee Health Science
Center, Campbell Clinic, Memphis,
Tennessee, USA

ALISTAIR YOUNGER, MB ChB, MSc, ChM,
FRCSC
Professor, Department of Orthopaedics,
University of British Columbia, Footbridge
Centre for Integrated Orthopaedic Care,
Vancouver, British Columbia, Canada

CONTENTS

Preface: Arthritis and Related Conditions   xv
Frederick M. Azar

Knee and Hip Reconstruction
Patrick C. Toy and William M. Mihalko

The Current Status of Cell-Based Therapies for Primary Knee Osteoarthritis   415
Rushabh M. Vakharia, Martin W. Roche, Jose Carlos Alcerro, and Carlos Jesus
Lavernia

There is a growing interest in utilizing cell therapy for treatment of knee osteoarthritis. The purpose of this study was to perform a systematic review on the current status of cell based therapies. The authors will review treatment modalities, clinical outcomes and the economics of cell therapy in the US.

A comprehensive literature search was performed on PubMED, Ovid MEDLINE, and Web of Science database from 1949 to 2019. The inclusion criteria consisted of articles containing cellular therapy, platelet-rich plasma, and knee osteoarthritis in the title of the manuscripts. Manuscripts which were letters, editorial material, abstracts not published, or manuscripts with incomplete data were excluded from the study.

Forty-two articles met our inclusion criteria and were critically reviewed by the authors.

Cell based therapy holds promise as a means of restoring local cartilage cell populations that are deficient due to injury or disease. These biological injectables, as a treatment for knee osteoarthritis, theoretically have potential but continue to be investigational.

At this time, there is no evidence-based information to justify the use of cell-based therapies in the treatment of knee osteoarthritis. In addition, the long-term effects of these modalities are yet to be determined.

Knee Osteoarthritis: Alternative Range of Motion Treatment   425
Rodney W. Benner, K. Donald Shelbourne, Scot N. Bauman, Adam Norris,
and Tinker Gray

Given the expected rise in the number of total knee arthroplasty (TKA) surgeries to soar to 3.5 million by 2030, an effective non-operative rehabilitation program is needed. Previous research at Shelbourne Knee Center taught us that any loss of normal knee extension (to include hyperextension) or flexion significantly affected subjective function. We began treating patients who had knee OA with a range of motion (ROM) based rehabilitation program that was delivered systematically, starting with ROM exercises for knee extension, followed by exercises for flexion and swelling reduction, before eventually starting a strengthening and conditioning program. In a group of 396 patients with knee OA, significant improvements were made in knee extension, flexion, and subjective scores for pain, symptoms, activities of daily living, sport, and quality of life. Furthermore, the ROM-based rehabilitation program prevented 76% of patients from undergoing TKA surgery.

Trauma
John C. Weinlein and Michael J. Beebe

Minimizing Posttraumatic Osteoarthritis After High-Energy Intra-Articular Fracture   433
Huai Ming Phen and Mara L. Schenker

This article serves to provide an overview of molecular and surgical interventions to minimize the progression of post traumatic arthritis following high energy intraarticular fractures. The roles of cartilage and the microcellular environment are discussed, as well as the response of the joint and cartilage to injury. Molecular therapies such as glucocorticoids, mesenchymal stem cells, and bisphosphonates are presented as potential treatments to prevent progression to posttraumatic arthritis. High energy intraarticular fractures of the elbow, hip, knee, and ankle are discussed, with emphasis on restoring anatomical alignment, articular reduction, and stability of the joint.

Posttraumatic Arthritis After Intra-Articular Distal Femur and Proximal Tibia Fractures   445
Jacob T. Davis and Matthew I. Rudloff

Posttraumatic Arthritis (PTA) is a form of joint degeneration that occurs after physical trauma to a synovial joint. Development of PTA is multifactorial and results from mechanical damage at the time of trauma, a cell mediated inflammatory response, and abnormal articulation due to persistent malalignment or joint instability. Though some risk factors may be unavoidable, preventing the development of PTA of the knee after intra-articular fracture (IAF) requires restoring anatomic articulation and alignment. Reconstruction with total knee arthroplasty (TKA) is the treatment of choice for PTA and may be a useful primary treatment for IAF in some.

Pediatrics
Jeffrey R. Sawyer and David D. Spence

Pediatric Septic Arthritis: An Update   461
Daniel W. Brown and Benjamin W. Sheffer

Septic arthritis in children is a surgical emergency and prompt diagnosis and treatment are mandatory. If diagnosed quickly and treated correctly, the outcomes can be good. With delay in diagnosis and without proper treatment, outcomes often are quite devastating, with growth disturbance and joint destruction.

Juvenile Idiopathic Arthritis for the Pediatric Orthopedic Surgeon   471
Karen M. Bovid and Mary D. Moore

Juvenile idiopathic arthritis includes conditions characterized by joint inflammation of unknown etiology lasting longer than 6 weeks in patients younger than 16 years. Diagnosis and medical management are complex and best coordinated by a pediatric rheumatologist. The mainstay of therapy is anti-inflammatory and biologic medications to control pain and joint inflammation. Orthopaedic surgical treatment may be indicated for deformity, limb length inequality, or end-stage arthritis. Evaluation of the cervical spine and appropriate medication management in consultation with the patient's rheumatologist are essential in perioperative care. Preoperative planning should take into account patient deformity, contracture, small size, osteopenia, and medical comorbidities.

Hand and Wrist
Benjamin M. Mauck and James H. Calandruccio

Arthritis of the Thumb Interphalangeal and Finger Distal Interphalangeal Joint   489
John C. Wu, James H. Calandruccio, William Jacob Weller, Peter R. Henning, and
Colin W. Swigler

> The DIP joints are subjected to the highest joint forces in the hand, and at least
> 60% of individuals older than age 60 years have DIP joint arthritis. Debridement
> of degenerative distal interphalandeal joints with mild to moderate disease can
> provide satisfactory outcomes; however, those joints with more severe angular
> and rotation changes are reliably treated with fusions. Regardless of the fixa-
> tion method, DIP fusions have high success rates, are well tolerated, and are
> extremely durable.

Evaluation and Management of Scaphoid-Trapezium-Trapezoid Joint Arthritis   497
John C. Wu and James H. Calandruccio

> Degenerative arthritis at the articulation of the scaphoid, trapezium, and trap-
> ezoid (STT or triscaphe joint) is a relatively common degenerative disease of
> the wrist. Pain and weakness with grip strength reduction and functional limita-
> tions when performing routine daily tasks such as opening a jar are common
> complaints of patients with STT arthritis. Initial conservative treatments for STT
> arthritis include splinting, bracing, activity modification, anti-inflammatory
> medication and steroid injections for pain relief. Failure of conservative treat-
> ment is the main indication for surgery, which may include distal scaphoid exci-
> sion, with or without filling of the void after excision, trapeziectomy, STT
> arthrodesis, or STT implant arthroplasty. Improvements in pain and motion
> have been reported with all of these techniques.

Shoulder and Elbow
Tyler J. Brolin

Management of the B2 Glenoid in Glenohumeral Osteoarthritis   509
Siddhant K. Mehta and Alexander W. Aleem

> The Walch B2 glenoid is characterized by a biconcave glenoid deformity, ac-
> quired glenoid retroversion, and posterior humeral head subluxation. Surgical
> reconstruction of the B2 glenoid remains a challenge. Surgical management
> options include arthroscopic debridement, hemiarthroplasty, anatomic total
> shoulder arthroplasty with eccentric reaming, bone grafting, or augmented
> glenoid implants, and reverse total shoulder arthroplasty. Multiple factors
> including patient age, level of activity, degree of glenoid retroversion, humeral
> head posterior subluxation, and rotator cuff integrity dictate the optimal surgi-
> cal management strategy. The surgeon must carefully consider these factors, as
> well as, take into account the relative advantages and disadvantages of each of
> these techniques to appropriately tailor a patient-specific surgical plan. This re-
> view article aims to describe each of these techniques and presents the current
> available literature in an effort to guide evidence-based decisions in the surgi-
> cal management of the B2 glenoid deformity.

Arthroscopic Management of Glenohumeral Arthritis   521
David C. Carver and Tyler J. Brolin

> Glenohumeral arthritis in the young adult is a particularly challenging condition
> for which optimal treatment algorithms have yet to be established. Arthro-
> scopic joint preserving treatments have the advantage of delaying arthroplasty
> in this younger population while maintaining the patient's natural anatomy and
> do not appear to compromise later arthroplasty. Various surgical techniques

are available such that the overall procedure is tailored to the patient's individual pathology. The majority of short- and mid-term studies show good outcomes with low conversion to total shoulder arthroplasty and sustained improvements in functional outcome scores.

Foot and Ankle
Clayton C. Bettin and Benjamin J. Grear

Pathogenesis of Posttraumatic Osteoarthritis of the Ankle   529
Eugene C. Nwankwo Jr, Lawal A. Labaran, Vincent Athas, Steve Olson,
and Samuel B. Adams

Ankle osteoarthritis affects a significant portion of the global adult population. Unlike other joints, arthritis of the ankle often develops as a response to traumatic injury (intra-articular fracture) of the ankle joints. The full mechanism leading to posttraumatic osteoarthritis of the ankle (PTOAA) is poorly understood. These deficits in knowledge pose challenges in the management of the disease. Adequate surgical reduction of fractured ankle joints remains the gold standard in preventing. The purpose of this review is to thoroughly delineate the known pathogenesis of PTOAA, and provide critical updates on this pathology and new avenues to provide therapeutic management of the disease.

Outcomes Following Total Ankle Arthroplasty: A Review of the Registry Data   539
and Current Literature
Luckshmana Jeyaseelan, Sam Si-Hyeong Park, Husam Al-Rumaih, Andrea Veljkovic,
Murray J. Penner, Kevin J. Wing, and Alistair Younger

End-stage ankle arthritis has a significant effect both on function and quality of life. Total ankle arthroplasty continues to emerge as a safe and effective treatment for ankle arthritis. With encouraging outcomes and improved implant longevity, there has been a significant improvement upon the results of the first-generation implants. This article reviews both the latest data from national registries and the wider literature to evaluate where we currently stand with outcomes of modern total ankle replacements.

ARTHRITIS AND RELATED CONDITIONS

FORTHCOMING ISSUES

January 2020
Reconstruction
Michael J. Beebe, Clayton C. Bettin, Tyler J.
Brolin, James H. Calandruccio, Benjamin J. Grear,
Benjamin M. Mauck, William M. Mihalko, Jeffrey R.
Sawyer, David D. Spence, Patrick C. Toy, and John
C. Weinlein, *Editors*

April 2020
Global Perspectives in Orthopedic Surgery
Michael J. Beebe, Clayton C. Bettin, Tyler J.
Brolin, James H. Calandruccio, Benjamin J. Grear,
Benjamin M. Mauck, William M. Mihalko, Jeffrey R.
Sawyer, David D. Spence, Patrick C. Toy, and John
C. Weinlein, *Editors*

July 2020
Minimally Invasive Surgery
Michael J. Beebe, Clayton C. Bettin, Tyler J.
Brolin, James H. Calandruccio, Benjamin J. Grear,
Benjamin M. Mauck, William M. Mihalko, Jeffrey R.
Sawyer, David D. Spence, Patrick C. Toy, and John
C. Weinlein, *Editors*

RECENT ISSUES

July 2019
Unique or Select Procedures
Michael J. Beebe, Clayton C. Bettin, Tyler J.
Brolin, James H. Calandruccio, Benjamin J. Grear,
Benjamin M. Mauck, William M. Mihalko, Jeffrey R.
Sawyer, Patrick C. Toy, and John C. Weinlein,
Editors

April 2019
Surgical Considerations for Osteoporosis,
Osteopenia, and Vitamin D Deficiency
Michael J. Beebe, Clayton C. Bettin, Tyler J.
Brolin, James H. Calandruccio, Benjamin J. Grear,
Benjamin M. Mauck, William M. Mihalko, Jeffrey R.
Sawyer, Patrick C. Toy, and John C. Weinlein,
Editors

January 2019
New Technologies
Michael J. Beebe, Clayton C. Bettin, Tyler J.
Brolin, James H. Calandruccio, Benjamin J. Grear,
Benjamin M. Mauck, William M. Mihalko, Jeffrey R.
Sawyer, Patrick C. Toy, and John C. Weinlein,
Editors

PREFACE

Arthritis and Related Conditions

Despite ongoing research and development of new treatment modalities, arthritis remains a serious health crisis in the United States. Recent estimates show that as many as 91 million Americans have arthritis (37%), including a third of those aged 18 to 64, plus an estimated 300,000 children. Arthritis is the leading cause of disability and earning loss among adults in the United States. The articles in this issue of *Orthopedic Clinics of North America* present information about causes and treatments in adults and children with arthritis.

The knee is the joint most frequently affected by osteoarthritis (OA), and Dr Vakharia and colleagues and Dr Benner and colleagues offer nonoperative options for its treatment. Critical review of the literature by Dr Vakharia and colleagues concerning treatment methods, clinical outcomes, and economics of cell-based therapy led them to conclude that currently there is no evidence-based information to justify the use of cell-based therapies in the treatment of knee OA. In an effort to reduce the number of total knee arthroplasties in patients with knee OA, Dr Benner and colleagues used a range-of-motion–based rehabilitation program in 396 patients and found that total knee arthroplasty was avoided in 76%.

As the causes of posttraumatic arthritis become better understood, so do methods to reduce its occurrence and improve treatment. Drs Phen and Schenker discuss molecular therapies, such as glucocorticoids, mesenchymal stem cells, and bisphosphonates, as potential treatments, and they emphasize restoration of anatomical alignment, articular reduction, and stability of the joint as important factors in preventing posttraumatic arthritis. These same factors are reiterated by Drs Davis and Rudloff in their discussion of arthritis after intraarticular femoral and proximal tibial fractures. Reconstruction with total knee arthroplasty is recommended for progressive posttraumatic arthritis and may be useful as primary treatment for some patients.

Septic arthritis in children is a surgical emergency for which prompt diagnosis and treatment are mandatory. Drs Brown and Sheffer emphasize the importance of accurate diagnosis and appropriate treatment in obtaining a good outcome.

They also point out that sometimes devastating sequelae, such as growth disturbance and joint destruction, occur when it is not recognized and treated promptly. Juvenile idiopathic arthritis is an entirely different type of arthritis in children and adolescents, with an unknown cause and often causing deformity and limb-length inequality. Drs Bovid and Moore discuss the importance of involving the child's rheumatologist in treatment choices and perioperative care.

The small joints of the hand and wrist are frequent targets of degenerative arthritis. More than 60% of individuals older than 60 years have distal interphalangeal joint arthritis, for which debridement may be adequate if involvement is mild to moderate. As noted by Dr Wu and colleagues, joints with more severe angular and rotation changes are reliably treated with fusions. Drs Wu and Calandruccio also present tips for diagnosis and treatment of scaphoid-trapezium-trapezoid (STT) joint arthritis. Initial conservative treatments for STT arthritis include splinting, bracing, activity modification, anti-inflammatory medication, and steroid injections for pain relief. Failure of conservative treatment is the main indication for surgery, which may include distal scaphoid excision, with or without filling of the void after excision, trapeziectomy, STT arthrodesis, or STT implant arthroplasty. Improvements in pain and motion have been reported with all of these techniques.

Drs Mehta and Aleem present surgical management options for glenohumeral arthritis, including arthroscopic debridement, hemiarthroplasty, anatomic total shoulder arthroplasty with eccentric reaming, bone grafting, or augmented glenoid implants, and reverse total shoulder arthroplasty; they describe the techniques as well as appropriate patient criteria for each. Drs Carver and Brolin describe arthroscopic techniques for management of glenohumeral arthritis and discuss the advantages of techniques that are tailored to the patient's individual pathologic condition.

The ankle is a frequent site of posttraumatic arthritis, especially after intraarticular fractures. Dr Nwankwo and colleagues emphasize the importance of adequate surgical reduction of

Orthop Clin N Am 50 (2019) xv–xvi
https://doi.org/10.1016/j.ocl.2019.06.005
0030-5898/19/© 2019 Published by Elsevier Inc.

these fractures. Their review thoroughly delineates the known pathogenesis of posttraumatic ankle OA and provides critical updates and new methods for therapeutic management. Total ankle arthroplasty is proving to be a safe and effect treatment for end-stage ankle arthritis. Dr Penner and colleagues review both the latest data from national registries and the wider literature to evaluate where we currently stand with outcomes of modern total ankle replacements.

With the ever-increasing number of patients with some type of arthritis (ranging from posttraumatic to idiopathic juvenile), it is imperative that we be informed about current methods of prevention and treatment. The authors in this issue have raised some interesting concepts and presented much useful information for orthopedic surgeons who treat these patients.

Frederick M. Azar, MD
University of Tennessee–Campbell Clinic
Department of Orthopaedic Surgery
1211 Union Avenue, Suite 510
Memphis, TN 38104, USA

E-mail address:
fazar@campbellclinic.com

Knee and Hip Reconstruction

The Current Status of Cell-Based Therapies for Primary Knee Osteoarthritis

Rushabh M. Vakharia, MD[a], Martin W. Roche, MD[a],
Jose Carlos Alcerro, MD[b,1], Carlos Jesus Lavernia, MD[c,*]

KEYWORDS

- Stem cells • Cell therapy • Conservative management • Knee osteoarthritis
- Platelet-rich plasma • PRP

KEY POINTS

- Cell-based therapy for the treatment of osteoarthritis lacks standardization with respect to the quantitative and qualitative characterization of the methods for cell harvest, processing, and transplantation/delivery.
- The US Food and Drug Administration's regulation of cell-based therapy for arthritis continues to be under scrutiny owing to efficacy and safety concerns.
- Well-conducted randomized clinical trials using cell-based therapies have been inconclusive, particularly in their ability to demonstrate efficacy with disease-modifying results.

INTRODUCTION

Osteoarthritis (OA) is a common disorder of the knee that affects individuals primarily as a result of cartilage degeneration. Increase in life expectancy has made this joint disease one of the leading sources of chronic pain and disability in the United States and other developed nations.[1] Nineteen percent of middle-aged adults suffer from the disease.[2] Its management continues to be the focus of many research efforts. Most of these efforts have been directed toward disease-modifying methods that could restore or reverse lost or damaged articular cartilage, provide pain relief, and increase function.[1-4] Among the nonsurgical treatment options for OA, the use of intraarticular injections of platelet-rich plasma (PRP) and stem cells have become quite popular. The use of cell-based therapies in medicine was introduced in the late 1960s as a way to modify disease processes. Its first application was in bone marrow transplantation for cancer.[3] These treatment modalities have a great potential and have resulted in the cure of some cancers. Some studies have also demonstrated the advantages to the use of PRP in wound healing and other soft tissue applications.[1-5] Etulain[5] found PRP to promote the revascularization of damaged tissue, restoration of damaged connective tissue, and proliferation and differentiation of mesenchymal stem cell into tissue-specific cell types.

Disclosure Statement: One of the authors (C.J. Lavernia) certifies that he has or may receive royalty payments or benefits in an amount of USD 10,000 to USD 100,000 from Stryker (Mahwah, NJ, USA). He also owns stock in Johnson & Johnson (New Brunswick, NJ, USA), Zimmer (Warsaw, IN, USA), Stryker (Mahwah, NJ, USA), Wright (Arlington, TN, USA), and Symmetry Medical (Warsaw, IN, USA).
The authors have received financial support from Arthritis Surgery & Research Foundation for this article.
[a] Holy Cross Hospital, Orthopedic Research Institute, 5597 North Dixie Highway, Fort Lauderdale, FL 33308, USA; [b] Orthopedic Surgery, Adult Joint Reconstruction, Instituto Hondureño de Seguridad Social, Tegucigalpa, Honduras; [c] Orthopedic Surgery, Adult Joint Reconstruction, Arthritis Surgery Research Foundation, Coral Gables, FL, USA
[1] Present address: Barrio La Granja No 202 - Tegucigalpa, Francisco Morazan, Honduras.
* Corresponding author. 2550 Southwest 37th Avenue #301, Coral Gables, FL 33134.
E-mail address: c@drlavernia.com

The development of stem cell-based and PRP therapy to treat OA continues to be an area of interest for many investigators.[4] The capability of stem cells to undergo self-renewal and multilineage differentiation, as well as having analgesic, immunomodulatory, and antiinflammatory properties, renders them as an attractive potential therapeutic agent for tissue repair.[6] Studies have sought to harness endogenous stem cells for regeneration and applying intraarticular injection of stem cells to stop the delay OA progression.

There is a paucity of evidence-based information in the literature on the current status of cell-based therapy treatments for patients with OA of the knee. Therefore, the purpose of this study was to:

1. Review and summarize the evidence-based information and the current status of cell-based therapies in the management of OA of the knee; and
2. Review some of the economics issues in these options for treating knee OA.

MATERIALS AND METHODS
Search Strategy
A review was performed using the Web of Science database in January of 2019, following the PRISMA guidelines. The searches were performed on PubMed, Ovid MEDLINE, and the Web of Science database from 1949 to 2019. Query terms for the study included were (Title = "knee osteoarthritis" AND Title = "cell therapy") used in combination for our search.

Inclusion and Exclusion Criteria
All articles on cell therapy for patients with knee OA were collated. From this result, the abstracts of resulting articles were reviewed by authors to determine which articles to exclude from the study. Letters, editorial material, abstracts not published, and manuscripts published in open-access journals were excluded from the study.

RESULTS

Forty-two articles met our inclusion criteria and were critically reviewed by the authors. Table 1 has a description of the articles that contained validated patient-oriented outcomes.

DISCUSSION

Currently used conservative measures, including self-management exercises, prescribed formal physical therapy programs, knee bracing, nonsteroidal antiinflammatory drugs (oral or

topical), narcotic medicine for refractory pain, and intraarticular injections of corticosteroids or hyaluronic acids (HAs), have been mostly unsuccessful in making significant changes in patients quality of life and changing the natural history of knee OA.[4] Most of these therapies offer limited improvements in quality of life at significant cost some with major side effects in some cases.[4]

Sources of Cell-Based Therapies
These newer cell-based injections could potentially provide a less invasive and less expensive alternative to surgery, and therefore represent a potentially attractive option for patients with articular cartilage lesions and OA.[7] Many cell-based techniques that claim cartilage repair or regeneration have been described with some encouraging results but at great cost and lacking evidence-based methodology. Some of these series report on a very small number of patients. All cell-based treatments use cells obtained from umbilical cord blood, fat deposits, peripheral blood, or bone marrow aspirates from the pelvis or knee. These cells are then processed with several types of devices and then injected into the knee joint. Recently the US Food and Drug Administration (FDA) provided legal guidance and only homologous "minimally manipulated tissue" can be used in these injections without government approval (see **Table 1**).

Current treatment modalities include the use of mesenchymal cells and platelets. Mesenchymal stem cells can be derived from umbilical blood, embryo (embryonic stem cells), or harvested from an adult. Embryonic stem cells are pluripotent and can morph into any cell type as well as replicate indefinitely.[7] Pluripotency distinguishes embryonic stem cells from adult stem cells; whereas embryonic stem cells can generate all cell types in the body, adult stem cells are multipotent and can produce only a limited number of cell types.[8] Adult stem cells are considered multipotent because their specialization potential is limited to 1 or more cell lines but not any tissue. The therapeutic potential of these adult stems cells is much more limited. According to some authors, adult fat stem cells are only able to turn into fat, liver stem cells can only turn into liver, and so on.[8] However, a multipotent stem cell known as a mesenchymal stem cell can give rise to several cell types. These multipotent stem cells can give rise to bone, muscle, cartilage, fat, and other similar tissues. Multipotent stem cells are thought to be found in most body organs, where they replace diseased or aged cells. Thus, they

Author, Year of Publication	Country	Sample Size	Injections Used	Outcomes Measured	Results
Table 1 **Studies included**					
Centeno et al,[19] 2008	USA	6	BM SC	VAS, WOMAC	VAS and WOMAC improvements
Pers et al,[20] 2016	France	18	AD SC	WOMAC	Significant improvements
Jo et al,[21] 2014	South Korea	18	AD SC	WOMAC	Significant improvements
Sekiya et al,[22] 2015	Japan	10	Synovial	Lysholm, Tegner Activity Levels	Improvements in Lysholm, but not Tegner
Koh et al,[23] 2015	South Korea	30	AD SC	KOOS, VAS, Lysholm	Significant improvements in all
Vega et al,[24] 2015	Spain	30	BM SC	VAS, WOMAC	Significant improvements in all
Koh & Choi,[25] 2012	South Korea	25	AD SC	Lysholm, Tegner, VAS	Improvements, but not Significant
Vangsness et al,[26] 2014	USA	55	MS	MRI, VAS	Significant improvements in All
Wong et al,[27] 2013	Singapore	56	BM SC	Tegner, Lysholm, MOCART	Significant improvements in all
Glynn et al,[28] 2018	Ireland	17	PRP	ICOAP, EUROQol, A/E	Significant improvements in ICOAP and EUROQol; no major AEs
Halpern et al,[29] 2013	US	37	PRP	MRI	No significant changes
Taniguchi et al,[30] 2018	Japan	10	PRP	A/E, VAS, JKOM	No AEs; significant improvements in VAS and JKOM
Cole et al,[31] 2017	USA	111	HA vs PRP	WOMAC, IKDC, Lysholm	No significant improvements
Raeissadat et al,[32] 2015	Iran	160	HA vs PRP	WOMAC	Significant improvement in PRP WOMAC
Patel et al,[33] 2013	India	78	PRP	WOMAC, VAS	Significant Improvements, but only for 6 mo
Dai et al,[34] 2017	China	1069	PRP	WOMAC, IKDC	Significant Improvements
Shen et al,[35] 2017	China	1423	PRP	WOMAC	Significant Improvements

Abbreviations: AD, adipose derived; AE, adverse events; BM, bone marrow; HA, hyaluronic acid; ICOAP, intermittent and constant osteoarthritis pain; IKDC, International Knee Documentation Committee; JKOM, Japanese Knee Osteoarthritis Measure; KOOS, Knee Injury and Osteoarthritis Outcome Score; MOCART, Magnetic Resonance Observation of Cartilage Repair Tissue; MS, mesenchymal; VAS, visual analog scale; WOMAC, Western Ontario and McMaster Osteoarthritis Index.

function to replenish the body's cells throughout an individual's life.[9] Mesenchymal stem cells of mesodermal origin have the capacity to differentiate into connective tissue. These cells can regenerate muscle, bone, cartilage, and tendon. Allogenic stem cells have potential immunogenicity and tumorgenicity, whereas homologous stem cells only have potential for tumorigenicity.

PRP is obtained by mechanical separation of the small solid components (red cells, white cells, and platelets) in human blood. Platelets play a role in homeostasis, through cell membrane adherence, aggregation, clot formation, and the release of substances that promote growth and tissue repair. Factors in the platelets influence the reactivity of blood vessels and blood cell types involved in angiogenesis and inflammation.[10] The platelet-obtained growth factors speed up the healing process, although the mechanism continues to be unclear. Concentration of these growth factors has been estimated to be 5 to 10 times greater when platelet are separated from the rest of the blood components through centrifugation.[11]

Stem Cell-Based Therapies

Several publications have reported limited trials using both manipulated and minimally manipulated cells. Manipulations of the cells include digestion with one of several types of enzymes, filtration, fractionation, and ex vivo culture. Minimal manipulations include centrifugation and mechanical fractionation.

Well-conducted randomized clinical trials using stem cells are scarce. Many of the published studies on stem cell therapy or PRP do not describe the harvesting methodology properly, are underpowered, and have a follow-up duration of less than 2 years.[12–18]

Centeno and associates[19] studied 6 female patients who were injected with bone marrow-derived mesenchymal stem cells. These patients all had grade IV Kellgren-Lawrence knee OA. These stem cells were injected after being cultured for 7 days. They reported that patients had significant improvements in patient-reported outcome measures, including visual analog scale (VAS) and the Western Ontario and McMaster Universities Arthritis Index (WOMAC) pain scores. Furthermore, patients also had improved function as assessed by walking distance to onset of pain and decreased patellar crepitus. Radiographic findings illustrated increased cartilage repair and decreased subchondral edema.[19]

Pers and colleagues[20] evaluated the efficacy of adipose derived mesenchymal stem cells in 18 patients with severe knee OA. The study divided the patients into 3 cohorts who were then treated with varying concentrations of adipose derived mesenchymal stem cells. Three different cell concentrations were used: a low (2×10^6 cells), medium (10×10^6 cells), and high (50×10^6 cells) number of cells. Primary outcomes analyzed included safety and efficacy. At the 6-month follow-up, the study demonstrated that their methodology was safe with no serious adverse events reported. They reported that patients being treated with low-dose adipose-derived mesenchymal stem cells had the most improvements. WOMAC scores (-33.1 ± 8.9; $P<.001$), VAS pain (-41.2 ± 13.3; $P<.05$), and the Knee Injury and Osteoarthritis Outcome Score

(31.8 ± 9.1; $P<.01$) improved the most when compared with medium and high concentrations of the adipose-derived mesenchymal stem cells.

In a similar study, 18 patients were injected with adipose-derived mesenchymal stem cells. Jo and colleagues[21] evaluated the impact of varying titrations of fat derived cells on WOMAC scores at the 6-month follow-up. Secondary outcomes included clinical, radiographic, arthroscopic, and histologic evaluations. Patients were equally distributed into low-dose (1.0×10^7), mid-dose (5×10^7) or high-dose (10×10^8) groups. They reported WOMAC scores improved significantly in the high-dose group, compared with the low-dose and mid-dose groups (54.2 ± 5.2–32.8 ± 6.3; $P = .003$). Additionally, arthroscopic findings showed large cartilage defects decreased approximately 47.5% ($P<.001$) in the high-dose group, but there were no significant changes in the other groups. Histologic evaluation demonstrated thick hyaline-like cartilage regeneration in the high-dose group with a glossy white matrix.

In a 3-year follow-up study, Sekiya and colleagues[22] investigated the effects of transplanting mesenchymal stem cells in 10 patients with cartilage defects on the femoral condyles. The main outcomes measured in the study were (1) MRI features, (2) histologic features, and (3) clinical evaluation scores in patients with cartilage defects. The results demonstrated that MRI score was 1.0 ± 0.3 before and 5.0 ± 0.7 after, and continued to increase after treatment in each patient ($P = .005$). Histologic analyses revealed improvement in the cartilage defects in each patient as measured by the Lysholm score, a 100-point scale used to determine knee function by measuring metrics such as knee instability, mechanical locking, and stair walking. The median score of all patients was 76 ± 7 before treatment compared with 95 ± 3 at the follow-up period, and increased after each treatments in each patient ($P = .005$).[22]

These findings by Sekiya and associates were reproducible by Koh and colleagues[23] when evaluating the impact of adipose-derived stem cells for knee OA in 30 patients. The primary outcomes measured included Knee Injury and Osteoarthritis Outcome Score, VAS, and Lysholm scores at the 3-month, 12-month, and 2-year follow-up visits. The study showed that clinical results significantly improved at the 2-year follow-up compared with the 12-month follow-up ($P<.05$). However, 5 patients demonstrated a higher Kellgren-Lawrence grade. On second look arthroscopy, 87.5% of elderly patients (14 of 16 patients), improved or maintained cartilage status 2-year postoperatively.

Vega and colleagues[24] compared the efficacy of allogenic bone marrow mesenchymal stem cells to HA. In a randomized trial of 30 patients (15 = stem cells; 15 = HA) clinical outcomes were followed for 1 year and included evaluating pain, disability, and quality of life. Additionally, articular cartilage quality was assessed by MRI. The results demonstrated that pain was significantly decreased at 6 and 12 months after stem cell transplantation, whereas patients treated with HA showed lesser improvements. Furthermore, the stem cell group had significant decreases at 6 and 12 months in the WOMAC and Lequesne scores compared with the HA group. Quantification of cartilage quality as assessed by MRI relaxation measurements showed significant decrease in poor cartilage areas, with cartilage quality improving in patients treated with stem cell therapy.

In a level III, therapeutic case-control study, Koh and Choi[25] evaluated the efficacy of mesenchymal stem cells isolated from the infrapatellar fat pad. Twenty-five patients were injected with 1.89×10^6 stem cells. Although the mean Lysholm, Tegner activity scale, and VAS scores of patients improved at the final follow-up visit, improvements in final scores were not statistically significant compared with the control cohorts. Additionally, the study showed there were no injection-related adverse events observed during the study interval. A major limitation to these studies is the small sample size, with an average sample size of 19.5 patients within all the collected studies.

In a multicenter randomized clinical trial study of 55 patients, Vangsness and colleagues[26] studied the effects of injecting adult human allogenic mesenchymal stem cells to the knee after partial medial meniscectomy. Patients were randomized into 3 treatment groups: group A (n = 18), receiving 50×10^6 allogenic mesenchymal stem cells; group B (n = 18), receiving 150×10^6 allogenic mesenchymal stem cells; and a control group (n = 19), receiving HA. Outcomes analyzed and assessed included meniscus regeneration, and patient-reported assessments at regular intervals for 2 years. At the final follow-up, they noted a total of 427 adverse events. Of the total adverse events, 272 were reported as mild, 126 as moderate, 27 as severe, and 1 as life-threatening. The most common adverse events were arthralgias, joint swelling, joint stiffness, injection site joint pain, joint effusion, headache, and peripheral edema. Comparing meniscal regeneration between the control group and groups A and B at various time intervals. The study demonstrated that at

the 6-month mark no statistically difference ($P = .535$), but statistically significant difference at the 12-month ($P = .022$) and 2-year ($P = .029$) marks. Patients with osteoarthritic changes who received mesenchymal stem cells experienced a significant reduction in pain scores (VAS) compared with controls. This trial studied patients immediately after meniscectomy. In addition, there were only 10 patients in each group and the follow-up was short.

In a prospective, randomized, controlled trial of 56 patients with a minimum 2 years of follow-up, Wong and colleagues[27] assessed the International Knee Documentation Committee (IKDC) score at 6 months, 1 year, and 2 years postoperatively. Secondary outcome measures were Tegner and Lysholm clinical scores and the 1-year postoperative Magnetic Resonance Observation of Cartilage Repair Tissue scores. These metrics are used to measure knee instability and severity of cartilage defects based on imaging, respectively. Patients were equally distributed within the study and control groups, receiving either cultured mesenchymal stem cells with HA 3 weeks after surgery or HA alone, respectively. Patients receiving stem cells showed an added improvement of all the patient-oriented outcomes measured. MRI scans performed at 1 year showed significant improved in the cartilage present for the stem cell group.[27]

Platelet-Rich Plasma Therapies

Glynn and colleagues[28] performed a feasibility study in the primary care setting with 17 patients, of which 14 were eligible to participate. Twelve patients were actually studied. Primary outcomes measured included total pain score, constant pain subscore, intermittent pain subscore, the EuroQol (EQ-5D-3 L) survey, and EQ-VAS scores. The study found at baseline 8 patients (67%) who reported being in constant pain. This number decreased to 2 patients reporting constant pain at follow-up. All 12 patients had total pain and intermittent pain scores of greater than zero at baseline. The mean self-rating of health utility patient-reported outcome measures increased from baseline to follow-up with a mean change of 10.8. Mean index values for also increased from baseline to final follow-up for a mean change of 0.32.

In a case series of 22 patients, Halpern and colleagues[29] reported on the use of PRP therapy for early knee OA. They reported a 56.2% decrease in mean baseline VAS pain scores at 6 months (from 4.06 to 1.78; $P<.001$). Fifteen patients underwent MRI assessment before and after PRP treatment, and 12 of the 15 patients demonstrated no significant worsening of OA in their patellofemoral joint. Additionally, there was no change in the appearance of OA 1 year after PRP therapy.

In a study performed in Japan, Taniguchi and colleagues[30] evaluated the effects of PRP injection for knee OA on VAS pain scores, Japanese Knee Osteoarthritis Measure and Japanese Orthopedic Association scores on 11 patients. The study found that minor adverse events were noted in all patients, but symptoms resolved within 48 hours after injection. The average VAS pain scores improved at the 6-month follow-up from 71.6 to 18.5 ($P<.05$), with 80% of patients having a decrease in VAS pain scores of 50% or more. Additionally, the average Japanese Knee Osteoarthritis Measure scores were 35.2 and 14.3 at baseline and at 1-month follow-up, respectively ($P<.05$).

In a large, randomized, controlled trial of 111 patients with symptomatic unilateral knee OA, Cole and colleagues[31] compared outcomes and the effects of PRP (n = 49) with HA (n = 50). The study assessed several metrics, including the WOMAC pain subscale, IKDC knee evaluation, VAS pain score, Lysholm knee score, and differences in intraarticular biochemical marker concentrations. The study found no difference between the cohorts with WOMAC pain scores; however, the study did find higher IKDC scores in the PRP group compared with HA at 24 weeks (65.5 vs 55.8; $P = .013$). Additionally, the PRP group had statistically lower VAS scores at 24 weeks (34.6 vs 48.6; $P = .009$). In the biochemical analysis, differences between groups approached significance for IL-1β (0.14 vs 0.34; $P = .05$) and tumor necrosis factor alpha (0.08 vs 0.2; $P = .06$) at the 12-week follow-up. The clinical significance of these improvements remains controversial.

Raeissadat and colleagues[32] also performed a randomized, clinical trial comparing the efficacy of PRP to HA in 160 patients (PRP = 87; HA = 73). All patients were prospectively evaluated before and at 12 month after treatments. Primary outcomes analyzed included the WOMAC and Short-Form 36 patient-reported outcome measures. The study found that, at the final 12-month follow-up, WOMAC scores were significantly improved in both groups, however better results were determined in the PRP group compared with the HA group ($P<.001$). Additionally, the study found that patients had greater improvements in patients with Kellgren-Lawrence OA score of 2.

In a prospective, double-blind, randomized, clinical trial, Patel and colleagues[33] compared

the efficacy of PRP to normal saline in 78 patients (156 knees). Patients were divided into 3 cohorts: group A (52 knees) received a single injection of PRP, group B (50 knees) received 2 injections of PRP 3 weeks apart, and group C (46 knees) received a single injection of normal saline. Clinical outcomes were evaluated using the WOMAC survey before treatment and at 6 weeks, 3 months, and 6 months after treatment. Pain was also assessed using the VAS survey. The study found significant improvements in all WOMAC parameters in group A and group B within 2 to 3 weeks and lasting until the final follow-up of 6 months. The mean WOMAC scores improved by approximately 50% from baseline to final follow-up in group A and group B, whereas for group C the WOMAC scores deteriorated from baseline. In conclusion, a single dose of white blood cell–filtered PRP in concentrations of 10 times the normal amount is effective as 2 injections to alleviate symptoms in early knee OA.

In a metaanalysis of all randomized clinical trials published, Dai and colleagues[34] found 10 trials with a total of 1069 patients. The analysis of the studies found that at 6 months after injection, PRP and HA had similar effects on pain relief and functional improvement. At 1 year after injection, PRP was associated with better pain relief based on WOMAC pain scores and functional improvement, based on WOMAC total score, IKDC, and the Lequesne score compared with HA. Additionally, the analysis by Dai and colleagues found that, compared with normal saline, PRP was more effective for pain relief by comparing WOMAC pain scores and functional improvement by assessing WOMAC function scores at 6 and 12 months after injection.

In another metaanalysis of 14 randomized, controlled trials including 1423 patients, Shen and colleagues[35] compared PRP with a control treatment, which included normal saline and HA. The follow-up ranged from 12 week to 1 year. Compared with the control group, PRP injections significantly decreased WOMAC pain subscores, WOMAC physical function subscores, and total WOMAC scores at 3, 6, and 12 months after injection. Additionally, PRP did not significantly increase the risk of postinjection adverse events.

Garay-Mendoza and coworkers[12] studied the effects of bone marrow stem cells in patients with knee OA, but only had 30 patients enrolled in the study (7 male; 23 female) with a follow-up period of 6 months. Similarly, Lamo-Espinosa and associates evaluated culture-expanded bone marrow stem cells in 20 patients (12 male; 8 female) with a follow-up period of 1 year.[13] Nguyen and colleagues[14] investigated the efficacy of PRP in 15 patients (3 males; 12 females) for a follow-up duration of 18 months. In another underpowered study Bansal and colleagues[15] assessed the efficacy of PRP use in 10 patients (3 males; 7 females). Wei and colleagues[16] investigated the use of bone marrow stem cells in 23 patients (17 males; 6 females) with knee OA with a 12-month follow-up period. Similarly, Shapiro and colleagues[17] also observed the effects of bone marrow stem cell use in knee OA in 25 patients (7 males; 18 females) with a follow-up period of 6 months.

A review on currently offered biological therapies promoted for articular cartilage defects and OA of the knee at leading arthroscopy and sports medicine conferences reported that 65% of the methodologies did not have any peer-reviewed clinical data supporting their use.[18]

Regulatory Environment

The FDA regulates cell therapies under section 361 of the Public Health Service Act. Only human homologous cellular and tissue products that are minimally manipulated are allowed in clinical practice and do not require formal FDA approval.[36] Minimal manipulation implies that the inherent biological nature or structure of the material has not been altered significantly. This implies that the safety profile of the resulting product is ensured.[36] Growing cartilage cells in the laboratory and transplanting or using allogenic applications requires formal FDA approval.

Two cellular therapies dominate the cell therapy market: autologous and allogeneic.[37] The purity of the cell or tissue product to be transplanted is paramount for safety, and the type and potency of the cells or tissues are important factors with respect to efficacy. In contrast with pharmaceutical products, which can be analyzed and identified at the end of the manufacturing process with the use of chemical analyses, information about the history of the cells in the stem cell–based product, the expression pattern of identifying markers, and the function of the cells are harder to asses and will all play a role in determining the type of stem cells and the purity and potency of the product. Although autologous stem cells are thought to be safe, they could potentially lead to undesired transformations.[38]

Cost

Most insurance companies do not cover these therapies. As a result, they have become a significant cash source for practices. These therapeutic interventions with little evidence based data to back their use provide substantial remuneration at a rate of approximately $900 for a PRP injection and $3000 for a stem cell injection.[4] The cost of the kits used in the preparation of these therapies are listed in **Table 2**, making them cash transactions with large profit margins. In 2017, a Medicare outpatient visit in our region (MAC 0910204) pays the surgeon $119.33 (CPT Code 99203) and an injection to a major joint reimburses $69.21 (CPT Code 20610).[4] As can be appreciated the margins for these unproven treatments are large. In addition the procedures are mostly paid for in cash.

Table 2
Comparison of PRP kits by price, preparation time, and approximate concentration factor

Method	Method Description	Price ($USD)	Preparation (min)	Approximate Concentration Factor
CHUV	Table-top centrifuge	3.62	30	2–3
Cell Saver Based System	COM.TEC dechez Fesnius	175	20	4–5
Biomet System GPS II	Druker 755 Centrifuge	700	30	8
RegenLab	Standard	320	30	2–6
Cytomedix Angel	Computer-aided system	495	25	4–5
Autogel System	Cytomedix Centrifuge	325	1–2	2–4
Genesis CS	Drucker 755	1550	16	10
Harvest Smart Prep2	Harvest Prep	420	16	6–8

Abbreviation: $USD, United States dollars.
Adapted from Akhundov K, Pietramaggiori G, Waselle L, et al. Development of a cost-effective method for platelet-rich plasma (PRP) preparation for topical wound healing. Ann Burns Fire Disasters 2012;25(4):210; with permission.

In a prospective cross-sectional study, Piuzzi and colleagues[39] analyzed the cost of PRP in the United States by contacting 210 orthopedic centers that provide PRP treatments for knee OA. The study reported an average price of PRP injection was $714.15 (range, $380–$1390; standard deviation, ±$144.08). They reported that the states with the PRP injections with the highest cost of (>$800) were California, Connecticut Delaware, Maine, Maryland, Massachusetts, Nevada, Nebraska, New Hampshire, New Jersey, and North Carolina. States where PRP with the lowest mean priced included Kentucky, Mississippi, New Mexico, Pennsylvania, and Texas. In a cross-sectional economic study by Alcerro and Lavernia[4] the authors found the mean cost of PRP injection in South Florida to be $897 (range, $350–$1700).

In the current marketplace, there is a wide variability in the costs of PRP kits that are available for manipulating tissue. Kit prices range from $3.62 to $1550, with preparation times ranging from 1 to 2 minutes to 30 minutes (see **Table 2**).[40]

In a similar study, Piuzzi and colleagues[41] performed a prospective cross-sectional study of orthopedic centers in the United States to determine the mean cost of stem cell therapy. A total of 317 centers were contacted with a response rate of 86.11% (n = 273). The data demonstrated an average cost of $5156.43 (range, $1150–$12,000; standard deviation, ±$2445.61), States with the highest average cost of stem cell therapy treatment, greater than $7,000, for knee OA included]: Delaware, Maryland, and North Carolina. States with the lowest average amount for stem cell therapy, with an average cost of $3000 or less, for knee OA included Arizona, Arkansas, Georgia, Montana, Pennsylvania, and Tennessee.[41] When analyzing the cost of PRP injection in South Florida, Alcerro and colleagues[4] their study found a mean cost of $3100 (range, $1200–$6000) for stem cell therapy injection.

SUMMARY

Cell-based therapy holds promise as a means of restoring local cartilage cell populations that are deficient owing to injury or disease. These biological injectables as a treatment for knee OA theoretically have significant potential but continue to be investigational. At this time, there is no evidence-based information to justify the use of cell-based therapies in the treatment of knee OA. In addition, the long-term effects of these modalities are yet to be determined.

REFERENCES

1. Pitcher MH, Von Korff M, Bushnell MC, et al. Prevalence and profile of high-impact chronic pain in the United States. J Pain 2019;20(2): 146–60.
2. Wallace IJ, Worthington S, Felson DT, et al. Knee osteoarthritis has doubled in prevalence since the mid-20th century. Proc Natl Acad Sci U S A 2017; 114(35):9332–6.
3. Buckley RH. Transplantation of hematopoietic stem cells in human severe combined immunodeficiency: longterm outcomes. Immunol Res 2011; 49(1–3):25–43.
4. Alcerro JC, Lavernia CJ. Stem cells and platelet-rich plasma for knee osteoarthritis: prevalence and cost in South Florida. J Am Acad Orthop Surg 2018. https://doi.org/10.5435/JAAOS-D-18-00343.
5. Etulain J. Platelets in wound healing and regenerative medicine. Platelets 2018;29(6):556–68.
6. Hosseini S, Taghiyar L, Safari F, et al. Regenerative medicine applications of mesenchymal stem cells. Adv Exp Med Biol 2018;1089:115–41.
7. Maniar HH, Tawari AA, Suk M, et al. The current role of stem cells in orthopaedic surgery. Malays Orthop J 2015;9(3):1–7.
8. Akpancar S, Tatar O, Turgut H, et al. The current perspectives of stem cell therapy in orthopedic surgery. Arch Trauma Res 2016;5(4):e37976.
9. Feng H. Is stem cell therapy the future of orthopedics? Knee Surg Relat Res 2018;30(3):177–8.
10. Cole BJ, Seroyer ST, Filardo G, et al. Platelet-rich plasma: where are we now and where are we going? Sports Health 2010;2(3):203–10.
11. Im GI. Clinical use of stem cells in orthopaedics. Eur Cell Mater 2017;33:183–96.
12. Garay-Mendoza D, Villarreal-Martínez L, Garza-Bedolla A, et al. The effect of intra-articular injection of autologous bone marrow stem cells on pain and knee function in patients with osteoarthritis. Int J Rheum Dis 2018;21(1):140–7.
13. Lamo-Espinosa JM, Mora G, Blanco JF, et al. Intra-articular injection of two different doses of autologous bone marrow mesenchymal stem cells versus hyaluronic acid in the treatment of knee osteoarthritis: multicenter randomized controlled clinical trial (phase I/II). J Transl Med 2016;14(1):246.
14. Nguyen PD, Tran TD-X, Nguyen HT-N, et al. Comparative clinical observation of arthroscopic microfracture in the presence and absence of a stromal vascular fraction injection for osteoarthritis. Stem Cells Transl Med 2017;6(1):187–95.
15. Bansal H, Comella K, Leon J, et al. Intra-articular injection in the knee of adipose derived stromal cells (stromal vascular fraction) and platelet rich plasma for osteoarthritis. J Transl Med 2017; 15(1):141.

16. Available at: http://www.jrnlappliedresearch.com/articles/Vol11Iss1/Vol11%20Iss1Wei.pdf. Accessed March 4, 2019.

17. Shapiro SA, Kazmerchak SE, Heckman MG, et al. A prospective, single-blind, placebo-controlled trial of bone marrow aspirate concentrate for knee osteoarthritis. Am J Sports Med 2017;45(1):82–90.

18. Hadley CJ, Shi WJ, Murphy H, et al. The clinical evidence behind biologic therapies promoted at annual orthopaedic meetings: a systematic review. Arthroscopy 2019;35(1):251–9.

19. Centeno CJ, Busse D, Kisiday J, et al. Increased knee cartilage volume in degenerative joint disease using percutaneously implanted, autologous mesenchymal stem cells. Pain Physician 2008;11(3):343–53.

20. Pers Y-M, Rackwitz L, Ferreira R, et al. Adipose mesenchymal stromal cell-based therapy for severe osteoarthritis of the knee: a phase I dose-escalation trial. Stem Cells Transl Med 2016;5(7):847–56.

21. Jo CH, Lee YG, Shin WH, et al. Intra-articular injection of mesenchymal stem cells for the treatment of osteoarthritis of the knee: a proof-of-concept clinical trial. Stem Cells 2014;32(5):1254–66.

22. Sekiya I, Muneta T, Horie M, et al. Arthroscopic transplantation of synovial stem cells improves clinical outcomes in knees with cartilage defects. Clin Orthop Relat Res 2015;473(7):2316–26.

23. Koh Y-G, Choi Y-J, Kwon S-K, et al. Clinical results and second-look arthroscopic findings after treatment with adipose-derived stem cells for knee osteoarthritis. Knee Surg Sports Traumatol Arthrosc 2015;23(5):1308–16.

24. Vega A, Martín-Ferrero MA, Del Canto F, et al. Treatment of knee osteoarthritis with allogeneic bone marrow mesenchymal stem cells: a randomized controlled trial. Transplantation 2015;99(8):1681–90.

25. Koh Y-G, Choi Y-J. Infrapatellar fat pad-derived mesenchymal stem cell therapy for knee osteoarthritis. Knee 2012;19(6):902–7.

26. Vangsness CT, Farr J, Boyd J, et al. Adult human mesenchymal stem cells delivered via intra-articular injection to the knee following partial medial meniscectomy: a randomized, double-blind, controlled study. J Bone Joint Surg Am 2014;96(2):90–8.

27. Wong KL, Lee KBL, Tai BC, et al. Injectable cultured bone marrow-derived mesenchymal stem cells in varus knees with cartilage defects undergoing high tibial osteotomy: a prospective, randomized controlled clinical trial with 2 years' follow-up. Arthroscopy 2013;29(12):2020–8.

28. Glynn LG, Mustafa A, Casey M, et al. Platelet-rich plasma (PRP) therapy for knee arthritis: a feasibility study in primary care. Pilot Feasibility Stud 2018;4:93.

29. Halpern B, Chaudhury S, Rodeo SA, et al. Clinical and MRI outcomes after platelet-rich plasma treatment for knee osteoarthritis. Clin J Sport Med 2013;23(3):238–9.

30. Taniguchi Y, Yoshioka T, Kanamori A, et al. Intra-articular platelet-rich plasma (PRP) injections for treating knee pain associated with osteoarthritis of the knee in the Japanese population: a phase I and IIa clinical trial. Nagoya J Med Sci 2018;80(1):39–51.

31. Cole BJ, Karas V, Hussey K, et al. Hyaluronic acid versus platelet-rich plasma: a prospective, double-blind randomized controlled trial comparing clinical outcomes and effects on intra-articular biology for the treatment of knee osteoarthritis. Am J Sports Med 2017;45(2):339–46.

32. Raeissadat SA, Rayegani SM, Hassanabadi H, et al. Knee osteoarthritis injection choices: platelet-rich plasma (PRP) versus hyaluronic acid (a one-year randomized clinical trial). Clin Med Insights Arthritis Musculoskelet Disord 2015;8:1–8.

33. Patel S, Dhillon MS, Aggarwal S, et al. Treatment with platelet-rich plasma is more effective than placebo for knee osteoarthritis: a prospective, double-blind, randomized trial. Am J Sports Med 2013;41(2):356–64.

34. Dai W-L, Zhou A-G, Zhang H, et al. Efficacy of platelet-rich plasma in the treatment of knee osteoarthritis: a meta-analysis of randomized controlled trials. Arthroscopy 2017;33(3):659–70.e1.

35. Shen L, Yuan T, Chen S, et al. The temporal effect of platelet-rich plasma on pain and physical function in the treatment of knee osteoarthritis: systematic review and meta-analysis of randomized controlled trials. J Orthop Surg Res 2017;12(1):16.

36. Knoepfler PS. From bench to FDA to bedside: US regulatory trends for new stem cell therapies. Adv Drug Deliv Rev 2015;82-83:192–6.

37. Halme DG, Kessler DA. FDA regulation of stem-cell-based therapies. N Engl J Med 2006;355(16):1730–5.

38. McLean K, Gong Y, Choi Y, et al. Human ovarian carcinoma–associated mesenchymal stem cells regulate cancer stem cells and tumorigenesis via altered BMP production. J Clin Invest 2011;121(8):3206–19.

39. Piuzzi NS, Ng M, Kantor A, et al. What Is the Price and Claimed Efficacy of Platelet-Rich Plasma Injections for the Treatment of Knee Osteoarthritis in the United States? J Knee Surg 2018. https://doi.org/10.1055/s-0038-1669953.

40. Akhundov K, Pietramaggiori G, Waselle L, et al. Development of a cost-effective method for platelet-rich plasma (PRP) preparation for topical wound healing. Ann Burns Fire Disasters 2012;25(4):207–13.

41. Piuzzi NS, Ng M, Chughtai M, et al. The stem-cell market for the treatment of knee osteoarthritis: a patient perspective. J Knee Surg 2018;31(6):551–6.

Knee Osteoarthritis
Alternative Range of Motion Treatment

Rodney W. Benner, MD*, K. Donald Shelbourne, MD,
Scot N. Bauman, PT, DPT, Adam Norris, Tinker Gray, MA

KEYWORDS

- Knee osteoarthritis • Range of motion • Rehabilitation • Total knee arthroplasty

---

KEY POINTS

- Full range of motion (ROM) in the knee is critical for optimal function. The opposite, normal knee must be examined to establish a baseline for normal ROM.
- Most nonoperative rehabilitation programs for knee osteoarthritis (OA) concentrate on increasing strength, which is difficult to achieve when any ROM loss is present.
- Total knee arthroplasty (TKA) surgery is expected to increase drastically, and an effective nonoperative rehabilitation program is needed to relieve symptoms for patients.
- The Shelbourne Knee Center ROM-based rehabilitation program emphasizes normalizing knee extension (to include hyperextension) first, followed by improving flexion and then strength.
- This ROM-based rehabilitation program was effective for improving ROM, pain, symptoms, and function in patients with OA, and 76% were prevented from undergoing TKA surgery.

INTRODUCTION
Background of Rehabilitation for Osteoarthritis

Because of the increasing prevalence of osteoarthritis (OA) and total knee arthroplasty (TKA) surgeries in the near future, a conservative nonoperative treatment approach is needed. Treating patients conservatively with rehabilitation can improve outcomes as a standalone treatment or to be used to maximize objective measures before a TKA, ultimately leading to better results postoperatively.[1,2] This approach, however, is not just for patients who have radiographic indications for surgery because exercise therapy can lead to positive outcomes regardless of the severity of OA, allowing it to be used by a broader patient population.[3] Most of the previous studies evaluating exercise therapy as a form of nonsurgical treatment of knee OA have looked at a variety of categories. These forms of exercise include stretching for knee range of motion (ROM), aerobic training for cardiorespiratory fitness, resistance training for increasing muscle strength, and performance training for improving activities of daily living.[4,5] All forms of exercise have been shown to improve patient outcomes; however, not all studies have a standard and structured treatment plan for patients with knee OA. Having a systematic approach to treating OA will not only allow the patient to improve but also allow them to maintain their gains for long-term success. It has been shown that gains made in the early phase of rehabilitation can be maintained for up to 6 months after starting treatment before ultimately declining; thus, patients are encouraged to continue treatment beyond the 12-week recommendation.[6] Patient education is important because the individual needs to know how to maintain the gains they achieved by the time of discharge so as to prevent symptoms from returning.

Disclosure Statement: The authors have nothing to disclose related to the content of this article.
Shelbourne Knee Center at Community East Hospital, 1500 North Ritter Avenue, Indianapolis, IN 46219, USA
* Corresponding author.
E-mail address: RBenner@ecommunity.com

Orthop Clin N Am 50 (2019) 425–432
https://doi.org/10.1016/j.ocl.2019.05.001
0030-5898/19/© 2019 The Authors. Published by Elsevier Inc.

The authors' preferred nonsurgical treatment of knee OA has been developed based on years of experience treating patients with anterior cruciate ligament (ACL) tears. The senior author (K.D.S.) has performed greater than 6000 ACL reconstructions and has seen only knee patients since the late 1980s. Multiple publications from the authors' center have highlighted the vital role that knee ROM plays in the long-term outcome and development of OA after ACL surgery, with loss of knee extension, flexion, or both consistently leading to a higher incidence of OA.[7–9] Further experience with referral cases to the authors' office of arthrofibrosis after ACL surgery revealed that knee ROM could improve, even when present for long intervals of time.[10] Consequently, a treatment approach was developed to prevent and/or treat knee stiffness.

Current estimates of TKA volume are expected to soar by 673% to 3.5 million by 2030.[11] Consequently, the ability of current infrastructure to handle that volume increase is in question. Furthermore, TKA is far from a certain outcome, with multiple reports of TKA dissatisfaction ranging up to 10% to 30% and beyond.[12–14] The authors have some guidance with regard to the effect of ROM on TKA outcome. Findings from Ritter and colleagues[15] revealed that knee ROM before TKA surgery will dictate postoperative ROM, and greater ROM has a positive impact on TKA outcomes.[16] If preoperative ROM dictates postoperative ROM and postoperative ROM directly influences outcome, it is thus imperative to maximize preoperative ROM before performing TKA surgery. In this way, the patient's chances of successful outcome can be modified and satisfaction maximized.

Initial Evaluation

At the authors' center, patients are seen by a physical therapist (PT) or athletic trainer (ATC) from the moment they enter the office. PT/ATCs serve as clinical assistants, whereby they take the patient's initial history, escort them to obtain radiographs, and then present the findings to the physician. The physician reviews the gathered information before entering the examination room, and both the physician and the PT/ATC evaluate the patient together. This arrangement provides connection and continuity between physician and therapy staff members to coordinate care. Once the physician completes the examination, the PT/ATC is able to listen to the physician/patient interaction, followed by immediately starting the therapy process dictated by the physician.

Radiographic evaluation is done to bilateral knees so side-to-side comparisons can be facilitated. Bilateral anteroposterior, 45° flexed weight-bearing posteroanterior, lateral, and Merchant views are obtained with in-house radiography. Joint space narrowing in all compartments, alignment, and ancillary changes are noted and reported in the medical record as well as reviewed with both the patient and the therapy provider.

Knee ROM assessment is done and reported in the record. Knee ROM is reported as 3 numbers a/b/c, with "a" being the degree of hyperextension, "b" being the degrees short of 0° neutral, and "c" being the degrees of flexion. A patient with 2° of hyperextension and 125° of flexion would be reported as 2/0/125°. A patient with 5° flexion contraction and 125° of flexion would be reported 0/5/125°. The normal knee (if present) is always measured first and serves as the standard of normal ROM. If both knees are involved, full extension is counted as any degree of hyperextension because almost all normal knees will achieve some.

Most studies do not include an evaluation of hyperextension and, instead, consider knee extension of 0° neutral as normal. A patient with 5° short of extension from neutral may not be considered to have much extension loss. However, if normal extension for that person is 5° of hyperextension, the flexion contracture is 10°.[17] DeCarlo and Sell[17] found that the mean degree of extension was 5° of hyperextension for men and 6° for women (Fig. 1). Several studies by Shelbourne and colleagues[7–9] found that even 3° loss of normal hyperextension resulted in lower subjective function scores and increased rate of developing OA in the long term after ACL reconstruction. Loss of normal

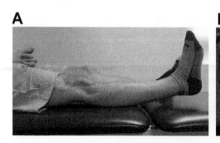
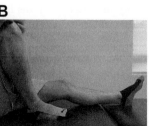

Fig. 1. The patient's right knee has 8° of hyperextension that is normal for him (A). His left knee shows 13° short of 0° neutral (B). The difference between knees is 21°.

knee extension can cause patients to limp and favor the noninvolved knee with standing and everyday activities of getting up from a chair and climbing stairs. The lack of normal use in the knee perpetuates the problem of loss of knee motion and can make it worse over time, and the patient develops a deconditioned knee. A deconditioned knee is defined as a painful syndrome caused by anatomic or functional abnormalities that result in a knee flexion contracture, functional loss of knee extension, decreased strength, and decreased function.[5] The authors have found that restoring normal knee extension or hyperextension (when present) is the key to reducing symptoms for patients.

When a patient with knee OA is found to have ROM deficits, the authors routinely prescribe physical therapy to restore or maximize ROM improvement before they consider TKA surgery. Nonsteroidal anti-inflammatories, intraarticular steroid injections, oral steroid dose packs, and light analgesics are prescribed by physician discretion.

SHELBOURNE KNEE CENTER APPROACH TO REHABILITATION
Philosophy of Range of Motion–Based Rehabilitation Protocol
Once the patient is evaluated by the orthopedic surgeon, diagnosed with OA, and deemed appropriate for conservative treatment, they are referred to work with a knee rehabilitation specialist. In rehabilitation, the patient has specific goals set for improving function and decreasing pain by restoring normal ROM, decreasing joint effusion, and increasing lower-extremity strength. In patients with unilateral symptoms, the aim is to get the involved knee symmetric with the uninvolved knee in terms of ROM, swelling, and strength. In patients who have bilateral involvement, the goals remain the same; however, without knowing presymptom ROM and strength, the goals are geared more toward a general maximization of all objective measures, while still being focused on maintaining symmetry side to side. To meet these goals successfully, treatment is delivered systematically starting with ROM exercises for knee extension, followed by ROM exercises for flexion and swelling reduction, before eventually starting a strengthening and conditioning program. During each phase of the rehabilitation program, the focus stays on the current principle without progressing to the next step until that particular goal is met. For example, when working toward attaining full knee extension, the patient will not be working on flexion or strengthening exercises. This single-focus rehabilitation

approach allows for more predictable progression in each phase, which tends to lead to better short- and long-term success. Once the patient attains symmetric and maximized ROM into extension and flexion, minimal joint effusion, and adequate strength, improvement from a pain and functional standpoint is typically seen. From here, they can be transitioned to a maintenance program for long-term conservative management of their OA.

Knee Extension
The first step to improving the patient's function and pain is creating symmetric extension equal to the other knee. The authors' rehabilitation staff starts by giving the patient a few exercises, including a heel prop with or without weight, towel stretch, and the use of a knee extension device for home use. The heel prop is done with the patient in a long sitting position with their heel on a surface high enough to get the knee suspended in the air, subsequently allowing gravity to pull it into maximum extension (Fig. 2). This heel prop can be done with or without weight added on top of the knee to increase the force going into extension. The towel stretch exercise is also done in a long sitting position with a towel or stretch strap placed around the foot with 1 hand on the strap and the other hand on the distal quad, just superior to the patella (Fig. 3). The patient is instructed to apply pressure down with the hand on the distal quad while the other is pulling the strap toward the chest to maximum tolerance. Applying the pressure down while pulling the strap ensures the exercise is maximizing joint mobility instead of muscle flexibility, which will help reach full extension, including any degree of hyperextension. Two extension device products commonly used in rehabilitation include an

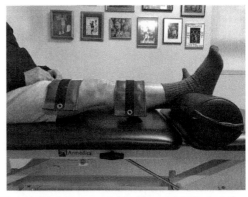

Fig. 2. Heel prop exercise. The patient is in a long sitting position with their heel on a surface high enough to get the knee suspended in the air, subsequently allowing gravity to pull it into maximum extension.

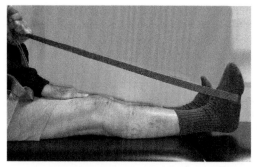

Fig. 3. Towel stretch exercise. The patient is in a long sitting position with a towel or stretch strap placed around the foot, 1 hand on the strap, and the other hand on the distal quad, just superior to the patella. The patient applies pressure down with the hand on the distal quad while the other pulls the strap toward the chest.

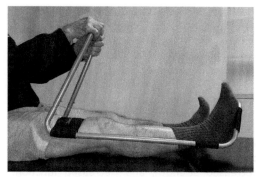

Fig. 5. The IdealKnee device. The patient places his or her leg in the device so that 1 strap is just above the knee and one is behind the ankle. The patient pulls back on the handle to bring the knee into maximum extension. (TS Ideal Products, LLC, Irvine, CA.)

Elite Seat (AKT Medical, Noblesville, IN, USA) and IdealKnee (IdealStretch, Park City, UT, USA). The Elite Seat is an extension device that places the patient lying supine with the involved leg elevated and heel propped up. Once in the setup position, 2 straps are placed across the knee both superior and inferior to the joint and firmly attached via a seatbelt mechanism. These straps are connected to a pulley system that is patient directed in terms of applying increasingly more force into extension for up to 10 minutes at a time (Fig. 4). By lying supine, the patient's hamstring muscles can be relaxed while applying pressure. The IdealKnee (Fig. 5) is a device that is used with the patient sitting with his or her legs extended. The device has a strap just above the knee and one behind the ankle that allow the patient to pull back on a handle to bring the knee into maximum extension.

The visit schedule for this stage of rehabilitation is roughly 1 visit every 1 to 2 weeks for ROM progression. In addition to the exercises given to the patient, they are encouraged to avoid favoring the noninvolved knee by purposely standing on the painful side, with the knee locked out into full extension. This standing habit not only maintains the gains made through the exercises but also starts creating a good habit of using the knee normally.

Knee Flexion

Once full extension is achieved, flexion exercises are started, such as heel slides, wall slides, and flexion hangs. Heel slides are done by the patient bringing the heel to the hip in a seated position and holding for a short period. Wall slides are done similarly, only that the patient lies supine with the involved foot placed on a wall, allowing gravity to bring the knee into a flexed position (Fig. 6). Flexion hangs are similar to the wall slides; instead, gravity brings the heel down without the

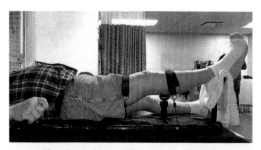

Fig. 4. Elite Seat device. The patient lies supine with the involved leg elevated and heel propped on the stirrup. Two straps are placed across the knee both superior and inferior to the joint and firmly attached via a seatbelt mechanism. These straps are connected to a pulley system that allows the patient to apply increasingly more force into extension for up to 10 minutes at a time. (Kneebourne Therapeutic, LLC, Noblesville, IN.)

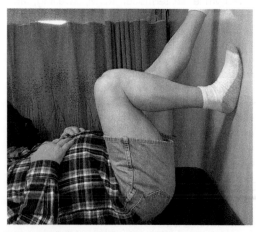

Fig. 6. Wall slide exercise. The patient lies supine with the involved foot placed on a wall. The patient gradually allows gravity to bring the knee into a flexed position.

aid of the wall, getting the knee into a flexed position to tolerance independently (Fig. 7). The visit schedule, like in the extension stage, is 1 visit every 1 to 2 weeks to assess and progress ROM. During this stage, the patient also uses cryotherapy, compression, and anti-inflammatory medication as needed to reduce swelling.

Low-Impact Conditioning

Once knee flexion will allow for a full and comfortable revolution on the bicycle or elliptical, low-impact conditioning commences. Performing conditioning exercises that are low impact in nature, such as biking, elliptical, swimming, or using a StairMaster, allows for light strength and conditioning gains without worry for acute flareups of pain or swelling that high-impact exercises would cause. Patients are encouraged to start a low-impact conditioning program every other day with minimal resistance, adding resistance and frequency as pain and swelling allow.

Strengthening

Once ROM and swelling are back to normal levels, strength is assessed unilaterally on both an isokinetic quadriceps strength test (Cybex) and an isometric single-leg press test. This assessment quantifies any deficit that they may have, making it easier to develop a strength program. The patient is given specific strength exercises to be done unilaterally to make up for the deficit that they have until they reach symmetry to within 10% of the contralateral side as measured on the isokinetic and single leg-press tests. Exercises used in this phase can be modified body weight exercises such as step-ups, step-downs, and single-leg partial squat or traditional gym exercises, such as single leg press, single knee extensions, and hamstring curls.

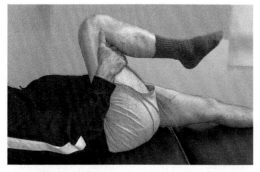

Fig. 7. Flexion hang exercise. The patient lies supine with the involved leg lifted in the air. The patient gradually relaxes their leg to allow the knee to bend, and gravity brings the heel down into a flexed position as tolerated.

The visit schedule during this stage is typically 1 visit every 4 to 8 weeks depending on the strength deficit to assess and progress their program. During this strength stage, the patient is still monitored for maintenance of adequate ROM and swelling, treating as needed. Once the patient is tested to be symmetric within 10% of the contralateral knee, a maintenance program is prescribed to continue treating the knee conservatively with rehabilitation long term.

Indications for Total Knee Arthroplasty Surgery

Progression to TKA is dictated by the patient's progress with the therapy protocol. Patients who make initial symptomatic improvements continue to follow-up with the PT/ATC until their goals are achieved, or a steady-state symptomatic plateau is achieved. Patients who are pleased with their progress and symptomatic improvement continue their home program on a maintenance basis. For those who are not pleased with their improvement, consultation with the surgeon is recommended by the PT/ATC, or by discussion with the treating surgeon.

Patients who have continued pain and symptoms are considered candidates for surgery if they have complete loss of joint space in at least 1 compartment. Rare cases of near-complete joint space loss are referred for surgery if they have not progressed or if they have moderate changes in multiple compartments. At this surgical consultation visit, the surgeon, therapist, and patient discuss the progress, or lack thereof, as well as the patient's expectations for their post-surgical outcome. Ideal candidates for a successful TKA are those who have made measureable functional gain with ROM and strength but continue to have pain. In this case, all are convinced that focused nonsurgical management has not been totally effective, that patient compliance is demonstrated by functional gains, and that pain relief that is reliably attained by TKA surgery will not be hindered by lack of full functional progression. Patients are asked to secure a caregiver for the first postoperative week; a preoperative talk and testing visit is scheduled; preoperative medical consultation by a hospitalist is sought, and a surgical date is selected.

RESULTS OF SHELBOURNE KNEE CENTER REHABILITATION PROTOCOL

The authors initially tested the effectiveness of their ROM-based protocol in 50 patients with deconditioned knees unilaterally.[5] The mean age of patients was 53.2 years, and 41 of 50 (82%) had a diagnosis of knee OA. Knee extension improved from a mean deficit between knees of 10° to 3° and flexion improved from a mean deficit of 19° to 9°. Patients had statistically significant improvements in both quadriceps muscle strength and subjective function. After some early anecdotal success with treating arthritic knees in this manner, in 2013, the authors began enrolling patients in a study to determine if these same symptomatic gains were possible specifically for patients with knee OA.

Between 2013 and 2017, 451 patients with knee OA and candidates for TKA surgery enrolled into a prospective study to determine whether the authors' ROM-based rehabilitation protocol could effectively improve knee ROM, reduce subjective symptoms, and prevent patients from undergoing a TKA surgery. Radiographs were graded in the medial, lateral, and patellofemoral compartments as mild, moderate, or severe according to International Knee Documentation Committee criteria. Mild OA was defined as minor detectable narrowing of joint space width or presence of small osteophytes and/or slight sclerosis or flattening of the femoral condyle. Moderate OA was defined as joint space width of 2 to 4 mm or narrowing up to 50%, and presence of sclerosis or osteophytes. Severe OA was defined as joint space of less than 2 mm or greater than 50% of joint space narrowing, and/or presence of large osteophytes. Knee ROM was measured consistently throughout rehabilitation and follow-up. Subjective function was evaluated at enrollment and at 1-, 3-, 6-, and 12-months follow-up with the Knee Injury and Osteoarthritis Outcome Score (KOOS) subjective survey, which evaluates pain, symptoms, activities of daily living, sport, and quality of life.

Fifty-five patients dropped out of the study, of which 11 had health issues, 2 died, and 42 dropped out for other reasons. Of the 396 remaining patients, there were 206 women and 190 men. The average age was 62 years old; 275 had unilateral knee symptoms, and 121 had bilateral symptoms.

Radiographic Grade

For patients with unilateral OA, the highest radiographic grade in any knee compartment was 48% severe, 33% moderate, and 19% mild. Patients with bilateral knee OA had more severe OA, with the highest grade of OA being severe in 69%, moderate in 17%, and mild in 14%. Bilateral OA patients also had more compartments in

their knees with OA, with 45% having 1 compartment involved, 40% having 2 compartments involved, and 13% having all 3 compartments involved, whereas patients with unilateral OA had 61% with 1 compartment involved, 33% had 2 compartments involved, and 6% had all 3 compartments involved.

Knee Range of Motion

The mean knee extension at enrollment was 4° short of 0° for both unilateral and bilateral knees; extension in the normal knee of unilateral patients was 2° of hyperextension. Significant improvement in mean extension was achieved by 1 month after treatment (4° for unilateral patients; 3° for both knees of bilateral patients) and was maintained through 1 year after treatment.

The mean knee flexion at enrollment was 117° for unilateral patients and 116° for the left knee and 117° for the right knee in bilateral patients. Knee flexion in the normal knee of unilateral patients was 131°. Statistically significant improvement in flexion was found in the unilateral group at 1 month after treatment and was maximized at 3 months at 128°. The improvement in the unilateral group was maintained through 1 year after treatment. For bilateral patients, mean knee flexion statistically significantly improved to 121° in both knees at 3 months after enrollment. Flexion was maintained through 6 months after enrollment but was found to be 117° at 1 year of follow-up.

Mean arc of motion was statistically significantly improved between enrollment and 1 month and was maintained through 1 year of follow-up (Table 1).

Knee Injury and Osteoarthritis Outcome Score Subjective Scores

Statistically significant improvement in KOOS scores was found for both the unilateral and the bilateral groups at 1 month after enrollment, and scores were maintained through 1 year of follow-up (Fig. 8).

Table 1
Mean arc of motion in the involved knees at enrollment and through follow-up after treatment

Group	At Enrollment	1 mo	3 mo	1 y
Unilateral	114	125[a]	128[a]	124[a]
Bilateral, left knee	112	118[a]	120[a]	116[a]
Bilateral, right knee	113	119[a]	120[a]	115[a]

[a] Significantly improved statistically from enrollment.

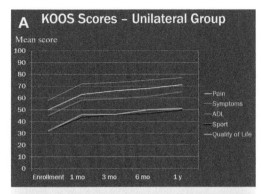

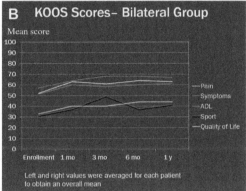

Fig. 8. Knee OA outcome score results for patients with (*A*) unilateral and (*B*) bilateral involvement. Scores show improvement in all categories between enrollment and 1 month after treatment; the scores are maintained through 1 year of follow-up. ADL, activities of daily living.

Subsequent Total Knee Arthroplasty Surgery
The purpose of providing the rehabilitation program was to improve patients' symptoms enough that they would not want to undergo TKA surgery. Of the 396 patients, 110 (24.4%) went on to undergo TKA surgery at a mean of 10.7 ± 7.1 (range 3.5–29 months after enrollment). The data of these patients up to the point when they had TKA surgery were included in the summary of results in this report.

DISCUSSION

The ROM-based rehabilitation program presented in this review has been effective and successful in the authors' practice for treating patients with a variety of knee conditions nonoperatively. Given the expected and alarming increase in the number of patients expected to undergo TKA surgery, the authors are encouraged by the success of the ROM-based program. The most important caveat of the program is that the clinician must evaluate for and recognize the patient's knee hyperextension

and then subsequently institute exercises to maximize its improvement before concentrating on other rehabilitation goals. Patient education of daily monitoring of ROM is also a key for long-term effectiveness. The principles of the rehabilitation are simple for patients to follow. If symptoms for the patient continue despite improvements in ROM, surgery can then be performed, and those improvements should yield better results with ROM after surgery.

SUMMARY

Full ROM in the knee is critical for any person to function at their highest level. Even a few degrees of extension or flexion loss can affect function and cause pain. The opposite, normal knee must be examined to establish a baseline for normal ROM. In patients with knee OA, most nonoperative rehabilitation programs concentrate on increasing strength, which is difficult to achieve when any ROM loss is present. The Shelbourne Knee Center ROM-based rehabilitation program emphasizes normalizing knee extension (to include hyperextension) first, followed by improving flexion and then strength. This ROM-based rehabilitation program has been effective for improving ROM, pain, symptoms, and function in patients with OA, and 76% were prevented from undergoing TKA surgery.

REFERENCES

1. Cross M, Smith E, Hoy D, et al. The global burden of hip and knee osteoarthritis: estimates from the global burden of disease 2010 study. Ann Rheum Dis 2014;73:1323–30.
2. Skou S, Pederson B, Abbott J, et al. Physical activity and exercise therapy benefit more than just symptoms and impairments in people with hip and knee osteoarthritis. J Orthop Sports Phys Ther 2018; 48(6):439–47.
3. Skou S, Deroshe C, Anderson M, et al. Nonoperative treatment improves pain irrespective of radiographic severity. A cohort study of 1,414 patients with knee osteoarthritis. Acta Orthop 2015;86: 599–604.
4. Juhl C, Christensen R, Roos E, et al. Impact of exercise type and dose on pain and disability on knee osteoarthritis: a systematic review and meta-regression analysis of randomized controlled trials. Arthritis Rheumatol 2014;66:622–36.
5. Shelbourne K, Biggs A, Gray T. Deconditioned knee: the effectiveness of a rehabilitation program that restores normal knee motion to improve symptoms and function. N Am J Sports Phys Ther 2007; 2(2):81–9.

6. Fransen M, McConnell S, Harmer A, et al. Exercise for osteoarthritis of the knee. Cochrane Database Syst Rev 2015;(1):CD004376.

7. Shelbourne KD, Benner RW, Gray T. Results of anterior cruciate ligament reconstruction with patellar tendon autografts. Objective factors associated with the development of osteoarthritis at 20 to 33 years after surgery. Am J Sports Med 2017;45:2730–8.

8. Shelbourne KD, Gray T. Minimum 10-year results after anterior cruciate ligament reconstruction: how the loss of normal knee motion compounds other factors related to the development of osteoarthritis after surgery. Am J Sports Med 2009;37:471–80.

9. Shelbourne KD, Urch SE, Gray T, et al. Loss of normal knee motion after anterior cruciate ligament reconstruction is associated with radiographic arthritic changes after surgery. Am J Sports Med 2012;40:108–13.

10. Shelbourne KD, Johnson GE. Outpatient surgical management of arthrofibrosis after anterior cruciate ligament surgery. Am J Sports Med 1994;22:192–7.

11. Kurtz S, Ong K, Lau E, et al. Projections of primary and revision hip and knee arthroplasty in the United States from 2005 and 2030. J Bone Joint Surg Am 2007;89:780–5.

12. Canovas F, Dagneaux L. Quality of life after total knee arthroplasty. Orthop Traumatol Surg Res 2018;104(1S):S41–6.

13. Kahlenberg CA, Nwachukwu BU, McLawhorn AS, et al. Patient satisfaction after total knee replacement: a systematic review. HSS J 2018;14:192–201.

14. Shan L, Shan B, Suzuki A, et al. Intermediate and long-term quality of life after total knee replacement. a systematic review and meta-analysis. J Bone Joint Surg Am 2015;97:156–68.

15. Ritter MA, Lutgring JD, Davis KE, et al. The role of flexion contracture on outcomes in primary total knee arthroplasty. J Arthoplasty 2007;22(8):1092–6.

16. Matsuda S, Kawahara S, Okazaki K, et al. Postoperative alignment and ROM affect patient satisfaction after TKA. Clin Orthop Relat Res 2013;47(1):127–33.

17. DeCarlo MS, Sell KE. Normative data for range of motion and single-leg hop in high school athletes. J Sport Rehabil 1997;6(3):246–55.

Trauma

Minimizing Posttraumatic Osteoarthritis After High-Energy Intra-Articular Fracture

Huai Ming Phen, MBBS*, Mara L. Schenker, MD[1]

KEYWORDS

- Posttraumatic • Osteoarthritis • Intra-articular • Incongruity • Malalignment • Instability

KEY POINTS

- Posttraumatic osteoarthritis predominantly affects younger patients. Arthroplasty in this population is limited due to longevity of implants.
- Intra-articular fracture results in acute chondral injury and subsequently changes the joint environment to hinder chondrocyte viability over the course of weeks.
- Few molecular therapies exist to augment the inflammatory and apoptotic environment following intra-articular fracture.
- Every joint is unique with regard to their dependence on stability, congruity, and alignment, making some more susceptible to posttraumatic arthritis.
- Articular reduction, joint stability and anatomic alignment are the cornerstones of treating high-energy intra-articular fractures to minimize progression to posttraumatic arthritis.

INTRODUCTION

High-energy intra-articular fractures are associated with the development of posttraumatic osteoarthritis (PTOA), a consequence that results in an estimated annual economic burden of approximately $3 billion within the United States and constitutes approximately 12% of all patients with osteoarthritis of the hip, knee, or ankle.[1]

Despite improvements in surgical technique and management of chondral injuries, the incidence of PTOA has remained relatively unchanged over the past few decades. Sustaining an articular fracture, by nature of the injury itself, can increase the risk of developing PTOA by up to 20-fold.[2–9] The 3 principal factors that influence the risk of developing PTOA following these fractures are thought to be joint incongruity, instability secondary to ligamentous disruption, and malalignment with abnormal loading of articular surfaces.

Given that PTOA can result in subjective impairment, chronic pain, and need for subsequent surgeries, clinical intervention to prevent progression toward PTOA is of paramount importance.[6,10] PTOA predominantly affects younger patients, and so arthroplasty in this cohort is limited by the life span of implants.[11,12] The pathogenesis of PTOA begins with the immediate chondral insult and local microcellular environment, and progresses to chronic cartilage overload as a result of incongruity or malalignment.

BIOLOGICAL RESPONSE TO HIGH-ENERGY INTRA-ARTICULAR FRACTURE

Articular Cartilage

Articular (hyaline) cartilage is a highly hydrated structure, composed of approximately 70% water held within a dense collagen extracellular matrix (types II, VI, IX, and XI), proteoglycans

---

Disclosure Statement: The authors have nothing to disclose.

Emory Orthopaedic Trauma & Fracture, 49 Jesse Hill Jr. Drive South East, 3rd Floor, Atlanta, GA 30303, USA

[1]Senior author

* Corresponding author.

E-mail address: hmphen@emory.edu

Orthop Clin N Am 50 (2019) 433–443

https://doi.org/10.1016/j.ocl.2019.05.002

0030-5898/19/Published by Elsevier Inc.

(aggrecan, decorin, biglycan, and fibromodulin), and chondrocytes. This unique and acellular structural composition serves to provide a painless articulating surface within a joint that is to function through strenuous, repetitive ranges of motion over a lifetime. This adaptation, however, results in a tissue that is inherently limited in its recovery capacity to traumatic injury. Cartilage may either recover or degrade following mechanical insult, with the latter resulting in PTOA.[13]

Acute Biological Response of Cartilaginous Injury

Chondrocyte death begins in the immediate phase following cartilaginous injury. Markers of apoptosis elevate (Box 1), altering the surrounding synovial fluid composition and resulting in chondrocyte necrosis and degradation over the course of weeks.[14–17] Cartilage explanted from patients sustaining intra-articular calcaneal fractures was significantly less viable than that from tissue donors who died of unrelated causes (73% vs 95%, $P = .005$).[18]

Articular Damage

Increased shear strain within chondrocytes is associated with a decrease in messenger RNA expression of aggrecan and collagen.[19] Incongruities within the articular surface affect the inherent biomechanics of the joint and disrupt the anatomic zones of contact, promoting internucleosomal DNA fragmentation within chondrocytes along with activation of caspases.[20–22]

Osseous Trauma

Repetitive mechanical injury to subchondral bone results in a surge of proinflammatory cytokines (interleukin [IL]-1, IL-6, tumor necrosis factor-α) and suppression of glycosaminoglycans.[23]

Box 1
Cartilaginous response to traumatic injury

Early Phase:

- Chondrocyte dysfunction and necrosis
- Degradation of extracellular matrix, reduced expression of messenger RNA components
- Elevated apoptotic markers, interleukin (IL)-1, IL-6, tumor necrosis factor-α, caspases, nitric oxide, reactive oxygen species

Late Phase:

- Osteoclastic activity promoting subchondral bone resorption
- Decreased expression of proteoglycans and glycosaminoglycans

---

Hemarthrosis from osseous bleeding is a potential contributor toward promoting expression of reactive oxygen species, elastase, and other lysosomal enzymes.[24] Subchondral damage results in increased osteoclastic activity, which may increase bone resorption and promote collapse of the articular surface.[22,25]

PHARMACOLOGIC THERAPIES

Despite the plethora of pharmacologic treatment options for established osteoarthritis, the gold standard of molecular intervention within the early stages of articular injury is still unclear. Treatment goals aim to attenuate the inflammatory response and its toxicity toward chondrocytes and to promote longevity and integrity of the articular surface.

Glucocorticoids

Corticosteroids, such as methylprednisolone, hydrocortisone, or dexamethasone, are commonly used adjuncts for treatment of osteoarthritis due to their anti-inflammatory properties. At low doses they are effective in treating symptoms; however, at higher concentrations they are associated with gross cartilage damage and chondrocyte toxicity.[26,27] In vitro and animal studies have shown that intra-articular dexamethasone injection soon after cartilaginous injury shows promise in mitigating the inflammatory response and promoting chondrocyte viability; however, further clinical information from randomized controlled trials with longer follow-up are needed to evaluate its clinical utility.[28–30]

Bisphosphonates

Bisphosphonates have been proposed to reduce the amount of peri-articular bone resorption.[31,32] High-dose versus low-dose alendronate therapy in a rodent model of periarticular fracture was shown to prevent early trabecular bone loss and cartilage degeneration at 14 days; however, at 56 days cartilage degeneration was seen uniformly regardless of dose.[32]

Hyaluronan

Hyaluronate supplementations are a widely accepted adjunct to the treatment of established osteoarthritis. High and low molecular weight hyaluronate intra-articular injections at day 7, 14, and 21 within a rodent model of induced osteochondral defects reduced cartilaginous apoptotic events and articular damage at day 28, but simultaneously promoted subacute synovitis.[33] A canine model study showed that serial intra-articular injections of hyaluronan versus saline control following anterior cruciate ligament (ACL) transection did not significantly alter the volume of synovial fluid or molecular weight of hyaluronan at 12 weeks, and the concentration of hyaluronan at this time was approximately 40% lower than that of preoperative values. The investigators concluded that intra-articular injections of hyaluronan do not supplement the quality of endogenous hyaluronic acid within synovial fluid; however, they postulated that a decreased proteoglycan level within hyaluronic acid–injected knees may have been secondary to analgesic benefit leading to increased activity levels.[34]

Mesenchymal Stem Cells
Mesenchymal stem cells (MSCs) have received much attention over the past decade for treating articular cartilage defects. They are often used as an adjunct to surgical interventions, such as microfracture or subchondral drilling; however, recent research has looked into their efficacy in isolation as well.[35,36] Chondrogenesis can be induced in vitro; however, this does not always translate to benefits in clinical application.[37,38] Intra-articular injection of MSCs within a rabbit model of osteochondral defects (OCDs) formed a fibrous tissue that covered the defect, but ultimately did not remodel into integrated hyaline cartilage. OCDs that were treated with direct local application of MSCs demonstrated a much more robust and abundant cartilage matrix, a thicker layer of regenerated cartilage that was similar to that of neighboring cartilage, and well-integrated borders between regenerated and native tissue as seen when stained with Toluidine blue.[39] In a similar study design, partial morphologic and histologic healing was observed 12 weeks postinjection within porcine models with OCDs of the femur.[40]

A randomized controlled double-blinded study looking into a therapeutic single injection of allogeneic MSCs and hyaluronic acid versus hyaluronic acid alone in patients undergoing ACL reconstruction demonstrated a greater joint space width increase at 18 months ($P = .03$) and 24 months ($P = .07$), along with an improvement in pain within the MSC and hyaluronic acid group, suggesting that more research may be appropriate to determine if these interventions result in long-term clinically relevant patient reported outcomes.[41]

CHRONIC JOINT OVERLOAD

Given that no pharmacologic therapy has been proven to arrest the development of PTOA, surgical management is still the current gold standard for these injuries. The goal is to establish an anatomic reduction and to introduce a fixation construct with absolute stability, to restore the articulating surface.

Finite element and experimental studies within cadaveric specimens have shown that joint incongruities can lead to contact stresses of up to 300% that of anatomic controls. Instability and increased contact stresses cause disproportionate increases in both contact stress rates and magnitudes, shifting the typical uniform, central location of joint loading to other areas.[42–45] This shift may be implicated in the progression of PTOA, as the new point of contact may be unable to accommodate physiologic load bearing.[46] Different joints exhibit individual tolerances to step-offs and instability (**Fig. 1**), and as such, the joints susceptible to *high-energy* intra-articular fractures are presented as follows.[47]

Elbow
A painless, mobile elbow joint is required to maintain independence with many activities of daily living such as feeding and personal hygiene. Its stability is conferred from primary, secondary, and dynamic stabilizers. Stiffness and pain following these injuries have been shown to reduce patients' quality of life.[48,49] Total elbow arthroplasty is the most definitive treatment for refractory osteoarthritis, but is generally considered a salvage procedure, especially in the younger population, largely due to the incidence of complications and failures from an increased demand in activity and longevity of the implants.

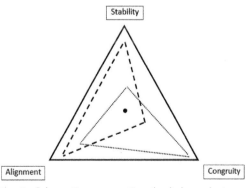

Fig. 1. Schematic representing the balance between congruity, stability, and alignment within articular joints. *Dotted line* represents an injured acetabulum. *Dashed line* represents an injured tibial plateau. Chronic cartilage injury affects the balance of joint congruity, stability, and alignment; however, this balance is *unique* to the joint in question.

Fractures of the distal humerus necessitate articular reduction, correction of rotation, and intensive rehabilitation following fixation with absolute stability constructs.[50] The trochleo-capitellar index (TCI) has been used in pediatric fractures of the distal humerus, and has been proposed as a method of evaluating the position of the capitellum and trochlea in relation to the humeral axis following surgical fixation to evaluate anatomic alignment and reduction. This study compared a triceps brachii elevating and olecranon osteotomy approach, using the TCI calculated from postoperative radiographs, with regard to Mayo Elbow Performance Score and range of motion. There was a positive correlation between TCI and better functional outcomes, but no significant difference between the 2 approaches.[51]

The efficacy of 4 intra-articular highly cross-linked hyaluronic acid derivative injections in patients with established PTOA of the elbow secondary to prior intra-articular fracture or dislocation has been investigated with respect to functional and pain-related outcomes. At 3 months, there was a slight improvement in Elbow Function Assessment Score of 1.47 points when compared with preinjection values, however at 6 months there was no statistical significance seen among all outcome measures. In this study, there was also no control group for comparison, and the time from injury was not assessed.[52]

The terrible triad injury includes a posterior ulno-humeral dislocation, radial head fracture, and coronoid fracture. Operative goals are to restore both stability and the articulating surface through lateral ligament reconstruction, coronoid fixation, and fixation/replacement of the radial head. Injury patterns associated with persistent joint instability include coronoid non-repair, medial collateral ligament injury, and radial head comminution.[53] Recurrent subluxation may occur in up to 8% to 45% of operative cases, and instability has been associated with a higher rate of second surgery and development of PTOA.[53,54] Delayed treatment of more than 2 weeks may be predictive of recurrent instability, and in this population, patients may benefit from temporary fixation before definitive surgery, with ulnohumeral cross pinning, external fixation, or internal joint stabilization.[54]

The coronoid process provides an anterior buttress within the normal arc of motion of the elbow; however, it may be difficult to achieve osteosynthesis for smaller type I or comminuted fractures. Although selected cases may be treated nonoperatively, a suture lasso technique using anchors for coronoid fixation has been described.[55,56] All patients within this series had concomitant radial head fixation or replacement, and lateral collateral ligament repair using nonabsorbable sutures and anchors, as well as a medial collateral ligament repair if instability persisted. The investigators found a lower implant failure rate with similar range of motion at 18 months, when compared with screw fixation.[57]

The radiocapitellar joint is a secondary stabilizer of the elbow, and an important constraint against valgus stress. Patients with an isolated radial head fracture treated nonoperatively with a minimum of 2-year follow-up showed negligible risk in the development of isolated radiocapitellar arthritis (0.1%).[58] Patients who progress to isolated radiocapitellar disease may benefit from radial head resection, partial interposition arthroplasty, or partial joint arthroplasty.[59]

Arthroscopic or open intervention for sequelae of intra-articular fractures of the elbow, such as impingement, loose bodies, or posttraumatic arthrofibrosis, has been described with generally favorable outcomes in terms of improvements in range of motion. Its indications, however, are still unclear due to the level of evidence of available and lack of long-term follow-up. Clinical judgment should be used when counseling patients preoperatively.[60–63]

Hip

The acetabulum is a hemispherical recess, formed by the triradiate cartilage between the ilium, ischium, and pubis, deepened by the peripheral labrum, lined with hyaline cartilage, and supported by its capsule. Articular reduction and internal fixation is the standard of care for displaced fractures. Total hip arthroplasty is indicated as a salvage procedure for symptoms refractory to further conservative measures.[64–66]

Restoration of the superior weight-bearing dome of the acetabulum decreases the rate of PTOA and improves clinical outcomes.[67] Posterior wall fractures have been shown to be a negative prognostic factor, suggesting this as a surrogate of instability and/or higher energy injuries. Cumulative survival of the native hip joint at 20 years in 810 patients treated surgically for acetabular fractures was 79%, and factors associated with need for total hip arthroplasty were posterior wall involvement, age older than 40, nonanatomical reduction, use of an extended iliofemoral approach, anterior dislocation, femoral head cartilage lesion, marginal impaction, and the initial displacement of the fracture greater than 20 mm.[68]

Computerized tomography (CT) has been shown to exhibit superior detection of gaps and step-offs compared with conventional imaging.[69,70] A study comparing plain radiography and CT after posterior wall fixation demonstrated that of the 65 patients with "anatomic" reductions on postoperative radiographs, 11 (17%) were found to have >2 mm of incongruities, and 52 (80%) had gapping of >2 mm.[71] A retrospective review of 227 patients followed for more than 2 years with postoperative CT scans found that gapping of more than 5 mm and an articular step-off of more than 1 mm were both independent predictors of conversion to total hip arthroplasty, suggesting that gapping is better tolerated than articular step-offs.[72] Intraoperative 3-dimensional (3D) imaging was found to improve postoperative articular incongruities by an average of 0.5 mm when compared with conventional fluoroscopic imaging; however, its utility may be offset by the presence of implants causing poor image quality.[73,74] Prospective trials with longer follow-up times are required before the use of 3D intraoperative imaging can be considered routine.[75]

Arthroscopy may be performed following high-energy dislocations to remove incarcerated fragments. A study looking into the utility of simultaneous hip arthroscopy before open reduction and internal fixation versus open reduction internal fixation alone did not show any difference in visual analog scale pain scores at 15 months.[76] Early surgical treatment within 7 days has also been associated as a protective factor in the development of PTOA; however, this was not found to be statistically significant.[77]

The quality of reduction has been shown to be imperative when fixing fractures of the acetabulum, whereas gapping of the fracture site seems to be better tolerated. Quality of reduction is best assessed with CT, which can allow for patient-centered discussions postoperatively regarding their prognosis.

Knee

High-energy periarticular injuries of the knee can result in residual malalignment and joint damage, progressing to PTOA in up to 45% of patients. Severe PTOA of the knee is salvaged with total knee arthroplasty; however, this is marred by an increased rate of revision surgery, infection, and other complications.[78–81] The gold standard for treatment of supracondylar femur fractures is that of articular reduction with absolute fixation, as well as implementation of fixation device that serves to minimize residual malalignment.[82–84]

The anterior and posterior cruciate ligaments, as well as the medial and lateral collateral ligaments serve to prevent excessive varus/valgus loading, as well as maintain anatomic rotation of the tibial plateau underneath the femoral condyles throughout dynamic weight bearing.[3] High-energy fractures of the tibial plateau are associated with meniscal or ligamentous injury in more than 50% of cases, with an increasing Schatzker grade of classification correlating with medial collateral ligament injury.[85,86]

Preoperative assessment with plain radiographs to assess the extent of injury in tibial plateau fractures was found to have poor interobserver reliability (±12 mm).[87] A cadaveric study investigating the interobserver accuracy of fluoroscopic reduction for tibial plateau fractures concluded that an anteroposterior and lateral view was adequate in detecting depressed fragments of 5 mm; however, direct visualization may be necessary to ensure malreduction of less than 5 mm.[5]

Preoperative CT scans allow for multiplanar visualization of fracture fragments, and predictions of soft tissue injury. A study reviewing preoperative CT scans of 132 patients with tibial plateau fractures showed that lateral depression greater than 11 mm was significantly associated with an increased risk of lateral meniscus tears. Medial tibial plateau displacement >3 mm, and fractures in a younger population with involvement of the anteromedial or posterolateral columns were found to be predictive of ACL avulsion fractures.[88]

Articular open reduction with internal fixation of bicondylar tibial plateau fractures provides the benefit of visualized anatomic reduction; however, limited internal fixation with circular frame application is also a viable option for patients with deficient soft tissue envelopes or when early weight bearing is desired, given its function as a load-sharing construct. Circular frames also offer the benefit of lower deep infection rates and fewer incidents of compartment syndrome; however, if malreduction is present in this setting, it has been shown to be predictive of PTOA.[8,9,89,90] It appears that the tibial plateau is able to tolerate larger articular step-offs than other joints, whereas instability or total meniscectomy are predictive in the development of PTOA.[91–94]

Arthroscopic-assisted fixation of tibial plateau fractures compared with traditional open techniques found that arthroscopy-assisted management was associated with a shorter hospital stay, decreased time to full weight bearing, and improved early range of motion, but long-term data were inconclusive, thus additional prospective studies would be of value.[95–97]

There is no consensus regarding how much incongruity is tolerated within the tibial plateau, with recommendations from 3 to 10 mm suggested. Joint stability, malalignment, and meniscal preservation have been more heavily and consistently implicated in progression toward PTOA, and as such, operative treatment should aim to restore all of these factors until controlled

studies that systematically evaluate these factors become available.

Ankle

In contrast to the hip and knee, primary talocrural arthritis is seldom seen, with PTOA being the most common etiology. Stability of the tibiotalar joint is conferred by the capsule, medial deltoid

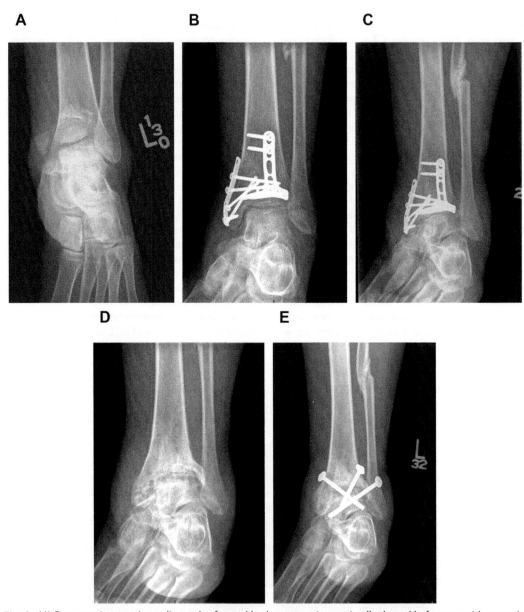

Fig. 2. (A) Preoperative mortise radiograph of an ankle demonstrating a trimalleolar ankle fracture with posterior subluxation (not shown). (B) Postoperative mortise radiograph of the ankle obtained 6 weeks after fracture fixation. Syndesmotic fixation was not required during intraoperative evaluation. (C) Postoperative mortise radiograph of the ankle at 10 months, showing progression to PTOA. (D) Radiograph following removal of hardware, better demonstrating the full progression to PTOA within 15 months of the initial injury. (E) Mortise view radiograph following arthrodesis that was performed for symptomatic control.

ligament, and lateral ligamentous structures. The syndesmotic structures stabilize the articulation between the distal tibia and fibula. Rotational ankle fractures, instability, and sprains were found to be the 3 most common causes of ankle PTOA in a consecutive series of 639 patients.[98] End-stage arthritis is treated with arthrodesis or total ankle replacement (Fig. 2).

High-energy axial loads through the tibial plafond result in pilon fractures, which have historically been difficult to treat due to the limited soft tissue envelope surrounding the fracture and the damage from compression across the articular surface during the initial injury.[3,99] Staged treatment of these injuries is advocated to minimize postoperative wound infection and trauma to the soft tissues.[100,101]

Surgical goals are restoration of native anatomic alignment, articular reduction, and prevention of chronic instability. Fibular fixation in pilon fractures is controversial. The benefit of indirect reduction of the Chaput and Volkmann fragments through restoration of fibular length is countered by the expense of wound healing and hardware complications, as well as increased construct stiffness, which may contribute to nonunion.[102] A retrospective study investigating 98 patients who sustained pilon and distal fibula fractures found that plate versus pin fixation of the fibula was associated with significantly improved reduction, and trended toward a lower rate of malunion and PTOA when compared with nonoperative management of the fibula.[103] A retrospective study of 93 patients undergoing fixation of the distal tibia either with or without fibular fixation found that postoperative alignment was similar between the 2 groups, and the only statistical finding between was the need for hardware removal.[104] Progression to PTOA was not evaluated.

Three-dimensional print-assisted surgery has been proposed as a method of improving intraoperative blood loss, reducing surgical times, and improving quality of reduction; however, the rates of PTOA were unchanged between the 2 treatment arms, and blinding was not uniform throughout any of the studies included.[105]

The optimal treatment of pilon fractures is still to be determined; however, staged treatment is advocated by many to minimize soft tissue trauma and allow for easier reduction at the time of fixation. Controlled, long-term studies investigating the variables contributing toward stability around the tibial plafond would be beneficial in ascertaining risk factors progressing to PTOA.

SUMMARY

Posttraumatic osteoarthritis following high-energy intra-articular fractures is multifactorial in its etiology, ranging from the immediate chondral insult to the long-term sequelae of malreduction, malalignment, or joint instability. Molecular studies are ongoing to identify and target the pathways responsible for chondrocyte necrosis in the peri-injury period, and may provide exciting therapies in the future that augment the cytokine cascade. The characteristics of individual joints seems to determine their ability to accommodate articular step-off or joint instability; however, the principles of operative fixation remain the same irrespective of this, obtaining as close to anatomic alignment, stability, and congruency as possible.

REFERENCES

1. Brown T, Johnston RC, Saltzman CL, et al. Posttraumatic osteoarthritis: a first estimate of incidence, prevalence, and burden of disease. J Orthop Trauma 2006;20(10):739–44.
2. Aurich M, Koenig V, Hofmann G. Comminuted intraarticular fractures of the tibial plateau lead to posttraumatic osteoarthritis of the knee: current treatment review. Asian J Surg 2018;41(2):99–105.
3. Beals TR, Harris R, Auston DA. Articular incongruity in the lower extremity: how much is too much? Orthop Clin North Am 2018;49(2):167–80.
4. Giannoudis PV, Tzioupis C, Papathanassopoulos A, et al. Articular step-off and risk of post-traumatic osteoarthritis. Evidence today. Injury 2010;41(10):986–95.
5. Haller JM, O'Toole R, Graves M, et al. How much articular displacement can be detected using fluoroscopy for tibial plateau fractures? Injury 2015;46(11):2243–7.
6. Marsh J, Weigel D, Dirschl D. Tibial plafond fractures: how do these ankles function over time? J Bone Joint Surg Am 2003;85(2):287–95.
7. Lutz M, Arora R, Krappinger D, et al. Arthritis predicting factors in distal intraarticular radius fractures. Arch Orthop Trauma Surg 2011;131(8):1121–6.
8. Thiagarajah S, Hancock GE, Mills EJ, et al. Malreduction of tibial articular width in bicondylar tibial plateau fractures treated with circular external fixation is associated with post-traumatic osteoarthritis. J Orthop 2019;16(1):91–6.
9. Weigel D, Marsh J. High-energy fractures of the tibial plateau: knee function after longer follow-up. J Bone Joint Surg Am 2002;84(9):1541–50.
10. Wasserstein D, Henry P, Paterson JM, et al. Risk of total knee arthroplasty after operatively treated

tibial plateau fracture: a matched-population-based cohort study. J Bone Joint Surg Am 2014; 96(2):144–50.

11. Roos E. Joint injury causes knee osteoarthritis in young adults. Curr Opin Rheumatol 2005;17: 195–200.

12. Hochberg M, Hochberg MC, Mead LA, et al. Joint injury in young adults and risk for subsequent knee and hip osteoarthritis. Ann Intern Med 2000;133:321–8.

13. Schenker ML, Mauck RL, Ahn J, et al. Pathogenesis and prevention of posttraumatic osteoarthritis after intra-articular fracture. J Am Acad Orthop Surg 2014;22(1):20–8.

14. Tew S, Kwan AP, Hann A, et al. The reactions of articular cartilage to experimental wounding: role of apoptosis. Arthritis Rheum 2000;43(1):215–25.

15. Catterall J, Stabler TV, Flannery CR, et al. Changes in serum and synovial fluid biomarkers after acute injury. Arthritis Res Ther 2010;12(6):R229.

16. D'Lima DD, Hashimoto S, Chen PC, et al. Human chondrocyte apoptosis in response to mechanical injury. Osteoarthritis Cartilage 2001;9(8):712–9.

17. Kim HT, Lo MY, Pillarisetty R. Chondrocyte apoptosis following intraarticular fracture in humans. Osteoarthritis Cartilage 2002;10(9):747–9.

18. Ball S, Jadin K, Allen RT, et al. Chondrocyte viability after intra-articular calcaneal fractures in humans. Foot Ankle Int 2007;28(6):665–8.

19. Ragan P, Badger AM, Cook M, et al. Down-regulation of chondrocyte aggrecan and type-IT collagen gene expression correlates with increases in static compression magnitude and duration. J Orthop Res 1999;17:836–42.

20. Islam N, Haqqi TM, Jepsen KJ, et al. Hydrostatic pressure induces apoptosis in human chondrocytes from osteoarthritic cartilage through up-regulation of tumor necrosis factor-alpha, inducible nitric oxide synthase, p53, c-myc, and bax-alpha, and suppression of bcl-2. J Cell Biochem 2002;87(3): 266–78.

21. Hashimoto S, Nishiyama T, Hayashi S, et al. Role of p53 in human chondrocyte apoptosis in response to shear strain. Arthritis Rheum 2009; 60(8):2340–9.

22. Pountos I, Giannoudis PV. Modulation of cartilage's response to injury: can chondrocyte apoptosis be reversed? Injury 2017;48(12):2657–69.

23. Lotz MK. Posttraumatic osteoarthritis: pathogenesis and pharmacological treatment options. Arthritis Res Ther 2010;12:211.

24. Borsiczky B, Fodor B, Rácz B, et al. Rapid leukocyte activation following intraarticular bleeding. J Orthop Res 2006;24(4):684–9.

25. Felson DT, Niu J, Neogi T, et al. Synovitis and the risk of knee osteoarthritis: the MOST Study. Osteoarthritis Cartilage 2016;24(3):458–64.

26. Xing W, Hao L, Yang X, et al. Glucocorticoids induce apoptosis by inhibiting microRNA cluster miR1792 expression in chondrocytic cells. Mol Med Rep 2014;10(2):881–6.

27. Wernecke C, Braun HJ, Dragoo JL. The effect of intra-articular corticosteroids on articular cartilage: a systematic review. Orthop J Sports Med 2015;3(5). 2325967115581163.

28. Huebner KD, Shrive NG, Frank CB. Dexamethasone inhibits inflammation and cartilage damage in a new model of post-traumatic osteoarthritis. J Orthop Res 2014;32(4):566–72.

29. Heard BJ, Barton KI, Chung M, et al. Single intra-articular dexamethasone injection immediately post-surgery in a rabbit model mitigates early inflammatory responses and post-traumatic osteoarthritis-like alterations. J Orthop Res 2015; 33(12):1826–34.

30. Grodzinsky AJ, Wang Y, Kakar S, et al. Intra-articular dexamethasone to inhibit the development of post-traumatic osteoarthritis. J Orthop Res 2017; 35(3):406–11.

31. MacNeil JA, Doschak MR, Zernicke RF, et al. Preservation of periarticular cancellous morphology and mechanical stiffness in post-traumatic experimental osteoarthritis by antiresorptive therapy. Clin Biomech (Bristol, Avon) 2008;23(3):365–71.

32. Khorasani MS, Diko S, Hsia AW, et al. Effect of alendronate on post-traumatic osteoarthritis induced by anterior cruciate ligament rupture in mice. Arthritis Res Ther 2015;17:30.

33. Galois L, Etienne S, Henrionnet C, et al. Ambivalent properties of hyaluronate and hylan during post-traumatic OA in the rat knee. Biomed Mater Eng 2011;22:235–42.

34. Smith GJ, Mickler EA, Myers SL, et al. Effect of intraarticular hyaluronan injection on synovial fluid hyaluronan in the early stage of canine post-traumatic osteoarthritis. J Rheumatol 2001;28(6): 1341–6.

35. McIlwraith CW, Frisbie DD, Rodkey WG, et al. Evaluation of intra-articular mesenchymal stem cells to augment healing of microfractured chondral defects. Arthroscopy 2011;27(11):1552–61.

36. Nam H, Karunanithi P, Loo WC, et al. The effects of staged intra-articular injection of cultured autologous mesenchymal stromal cells on the repair of damaged cartilage: a pilot study in caprine model. Arthritis Res Ther 2013;15.

37. Murdoch AD, Grady LM, Ablett MP, et al. Chondrogenic differentiation of human bone marrow stem cells in transwell cultures: generation of scaffold-free cartilage. Stem Cells 2007;25(11): 2786–96.

38. Pittenger M, Mackay AM, Beck SC, et al. Multilineage potential of adult human mesenchymal stem cells. Science 1999;284(5411):143–6.

39. Koga H, Shimaya M, Muneta T, et al. Local adherent technique for transplanting mesenchymal stem cells as a potential treatment of cartilage defect. Arthritis Res Ther 2008;10(4):R84.

40. Lee KB, Hui JH, Song IC, et al. Injectable mesenchymal stem cell therapy for large cartilage defects–a porcine model. Stem Cells 2007;25(11): 2964–71.

41. Wang Y, Shimmin A, Ghosh P, et al. Safety, tolerability, clinical, and joint structural outcomes of a single intra-articular injection of allogeneic mesenchymal precursor cells in patients following anterior cruciate ligament reconstruction: a controlled double-blind randomised trial. Arthritis Res Ther 2017;19(1):180.

42. McKinley T, Rudert MJ, Tochigi Y, et al. Incongruity-dependent changes of contact stress rates in human cadaveric ankles. J Orthop Trauma 2006; 20:732–73.

43. McKinley TO, Tochigi Y, Rudert MJ, et al. The effect of incongruity and instability on contact stress directional gradients in human cadaveric ankles. Osteoarthritis Cartilage 2008;16(11):1363–9.

44. Goreham-Voss CM, McKinley TO, Brown TD. A finite element exploration of cartilage stress near an articular incongruity during unstable motion. J Biomech 2007;40(15):3438–47.

45. Li W, Anderson DD, Goldsworthy JK, et al. Patient-specific finite element analysis of chronic contact stress exposure after intraarticular fracture of the tibial plafond. J Orthop Res 2008;26(8):1039–45.

46. Anderson DD, Van Hofwegen C, Marsh JL, et al. Is elevated contact stress predictive of posttraumatic osteoarthritis for imprecisely reduced tibial plafond fractures? J Orthop Res 2011;29(1): 33–9.

47. Novakofski KD, Berg LC, Bronzini I, et al. Joint-dependent response to impact and implications for post-traumatic osteoarthritis. Osteoarthritis Cartilage 2015;23(7):1130–7.

48. Biswas D, Wysocki RW, Cohen MS. Primary and posttraumatic arthritis of the elbow. Arthritis 2013;2013:473259.

49. Giannicola G, Bullitta G, Sacchetti FM, et al. Change in quality of life and cost/utility analysis in open stage-related surgical treatment of elbow stiffness. Orthopedics 2013;36(7):923–30.

50. Amir S, Jannis S, Daniel R. Distal humerus fractures: a review of current therapy concepts. Curr Rev Musculoskelet Med 2016;9(2):199–206.

51. Rollo G, Rotini R, Eygendaal D, et al. Effect of trochleocapitellar index on adult patient-reported outcomes after noncomminuted intra-articular distal humeral fractures. J Shoulder Elbow Surg 2018;27(7):1326–32.

52. van Brakel RW, Eygendaal D. Intra-articular injection of hyaluronic acid is not effective for the treatment of post-traumatic osteoarthritis of the elbow. Arthroscopy 2006;22(11):1199–203.

53. Jung SW, Kim DH, Kang SH, et al. Risk factors that influence subsequent recurrent instability in terrible triad injury of the elbow. J Orthop Trauma 2019;33(5):250–5.

54. Zhang D, Tarabochia M, Janssen S, et al. Risk of subluxation or dislocation after operative treatment of terrible triad injuries. J Orthop Trauma 2016;30(12):660–3.

55. Papatheodorou LK, Rubright JH, Heim KA, et al. Terrible triad injuries of the elbow: does the coronoid always need to be fixed? Clin Orthop Relat Res 2014;472(7):2084–91.

56. Najd Mazhar F, Jafari D, Mirzaei A. Evaluation of functional outcome after nonsurgical management of terrible triad injuries of the elbow. J Shoulder Elbow Surg 2017;26(8): 1342–7.

57. Garrigues GE, Wray WH 3rd, Lindenhovius AL, et al. Fixation of the coronoid process in elbow fracture-dislocations. J Bone Joint Surg Am 2011;93(20):1873–81.

58. Kachooei A, Ring D. Evaluation of radiocapitellar arthritis in patients with a second radiograph at least 2 years after nonoperative treatment of an isolated radial head fracture. Arch Bone Jt Surg 2017;5(6):375–9.

59. Sears BW, Puskas GJ, Morrey ME, et al. Posttraumatic elbow arthritis in the young adult: evaluation and management. J Am Acad Orthop Surg 2012;20(11):704–14.

60. Phillips B, Strasburger S. Arthroscopic treatment of arthrofibrosis of the elbow joint. Arthroscopy 1998;14(1):38–44.

61. Yeoh KM, King GJ, Faber KJ, et al. Evidence-based indications for elbow arthroscopy. Arthroscopy 2012;28(2):272–82.

62. Merolla G, Buononato C, Chillemi C, et al. Arthroscopic joint debridement and capsular release in primary and post-traumatic elbow osteoarthritis: a retrospective blinded cohort study with minimum 24-month follow-up. Musculoskelet Surg 2015;99:83–90.

63. Cikes M, Jolles B, Farron A. Open elbow arthrolysis for posttraumatic elbow stiffness. J Orthop Trauma 2006;20:405–9.

64. Matta J, Mehne D, Roffi R. Fractures of the acetabulum: early results of a prospective study. Clin Orthop Relat Res 1984;205:241–50.

65. Matta J, Merritt P. Displaced acetabular fractures. Clin Orthop Relat Res 1988;230:83–97.

66. Bhandari M, Matta J, Ferguson T, et al. Predictors of clinical and radiological outcome in patients with fractures of the acetabulum and concomitant posterior dislocation of the hip. J Bone Joint Surg Br 2006;88(12):1618–24.

67. Giannoudis P, Grotz MR, Papakostidis C, et al. Operative treatment of displaced fractures of the acetabulum: a meta-analysis. J Bone Joint Surg Br 2005;87(1):2–9.

68. Tannast M, Najibi S, Matta JM. Two to twenty-year survivorship of the hip in 810 patients with operatively treated acetabular fractures. J Bone Joint Surg Am 2012;94(17):1559–67.

69. Verbeek DO, van der List JP, Villa JC, et al. Postoperative CT is superior for acetabular fracture reduction assessment and reliably predicts hip survivorship. J Bone Joint Surg Am 2017;99(20): 1745–52.

70. Verbeek DO, van der List JP, Moloney GB, et al. Assessing postoperative reduction after acetabular fracture surgery: a standardized digital computed tomography-based method. J Orthop Trauma 2018;32(7):e284–8.

71. Moed B, Carr SE, Gruson KI, et al. Computed tomographic assessment of fractures of the posterior wall of the acetabulum after operative treatment. J Bone Joint Surg Am 2003;85-A(3):512–22.

72. Verbeek DO, van der List JP, Tissue CM, et al. Predictors for long-term hip survivorship following acetabular fracture surgery: importance of gap compared with step displacement. J Bone Joint Surg Am 2018;100(11):922–9.

73. Eckardt H, Lind D, Toendevold E. Open reduction and internal fixation aided by intraoperative 3-dimensional imaging improved the articular reduction in 72 displaced acetabular fractures. Acta Orthop 2015;86(6):684–9.

74. Keil H, Beisemann N, Schnetzke M, et al. Intraoperative assessment of reduction and implant placement in acetabular fractures-limitations of 3D-imaging compared to computed tomography. J Orthop Surg Res 2018;13(1):78.

75. Sebaaly A, Riouallon G, Zaraa M, et al. The added value of intraoperative CT scanner and screw navigation in displaced posterior wall acetabular fracture with articular impaction. Orthop Traumatol Surg Res 2016;102(7):947–50.

76. Kim HJ, Kim SS, Jung YH, et al. Effectiveness of hip arthroscopy performed simultaneously before open reduction and internal fixation for acetabular fracture and fracture-dislocation of the hip. Hip Pelvis 2018;30(2):92–100.

77. Cahueque M, Martínez M, Cobar A, et al. Early reduction of acetabular fractures decreases the risk of post-traumatic hip osteoarthritis? J Clin Orthop Trauma 2017;8(4):320–6.

78. Shearer DW, Chow V, Bozic KJ, et al. The predictors of outcome in total knee arthroplasty for post-traumatic arthritis. Knee 2013;20(6):432–6.

79. Houdek MT, Watts CD, Shannon SF, et al. Post-traumatic total knee arthroplasty continues to have worse outcome than total knee arthroplasty for osteoarthritis. J Arthroplasty 2016;31(1): 118–23.

80. Abdel MP, von Roth P, Cross WW, et al. Total knee arthroplasty in patients with a prior tibial plateau fracture: a long-term report at 15 years. J Arthroplasty 2015;30(12):2170–2.

81. El-Galaly A, Haldrup S, Pedersen AB, et al. Increased risk of early and medium-term revision after post-fracture total knee arthroplasty. Acta Orthop 2017;88(3):263–8.

82. Frigg R, Appenzeller A, Christensen R, et al. The development of the distal femur Less Invasive Stabilization System (LISS). Injury 2001;32:SC24–31.

83. Steinberg EL, Elis J, Steinberg Y, et al. A double-plating approach to distal femur fracture: a clinical study. Injury 2017;48(10):2260–5.

84. Kim JW, Oh CW, Oh JK, et al. Malalignment after minimally invasive plate osteosynthesis in distal femoral fractures. Injury 2017;48(3):751–7.

85. Stannard J, Lopez R, Volgas D. Soft tissue injury of the knee after tibial plateau fractures. J Knee Surg 2010;23(4):187–92.

86. Porrino J, Richardson ML, Hovis K, et al. Association of tibial plateau fracture morphology with ligament disruption in the context of multiligament knee injury. Curr Probl Diagn Radiol 2018;47(6): 410–6.

87. Martin J, Marsh JL, Nepola JV, et al. Radiographic fracture assessments: which ones can we reliably make? J Orthop Trauma 2000;14(6):379–85.

88. Tang HC, Chen IJ, Yeh YC, et al. Correlation of parameters on preoperative CT images with intra-articular soft-tissue injuries in acute tibial plateau fractures: a review of 132 patients receiving ARIF. Injury 2017;48(3):745–50.

89. Barei D, Nork SE, Mills WJ, et al. Functional outcomes of severe bicondylar tibial plateau fractures treated with dual incisions and medial and lateral plates. J Bone Joint Surg Am 2006;88:1713–21.

90. Canadian Orthopaedic Trauma Society. Open reduction and internal fixation compared with circular fixator application for bicondylar tibial plateau fractures. Results of a multicenter, prospective, randomized clinical trial. J Bone Joint Surg Am 2006;88(12):2613–23.

91. Manidakis N, Dosani A, Dimitriou R, et al. Tibial plateau fractures: functional outcome and incidence of osteoarthritis in 125 cases. Int Orthop 2010;34(4):565–70.

92. McKinley TO, Rudert MJ, Koos DC, et al. Incongruity versus instability in the etiology of posttraumatic arthritis. Clin Orthop Relat Res 2004;423: 44–51.

93. Rasmussen P. Tibial condylar fractures. Impairment of knee joint stability as an indication for surgical treatment. J Bone Joint Surg Am 1973;55(7): 1331–50.

94. Honkonen S. Indications for surgical treatment of tibial condyle fractures. Clin Orthop Relat Res 1994;302:199–205.

95. Fowble C, Zimmer J, Schepsis A. The role of arthroscopy in the assessment and treatment of tibial plateau fractures. Arthroscopy 1993;9(5): 584–90.

96. Ohdera T, Tokunaga M, Hiroshima S, et al. Arthroscopic management of tibial plateau fractures: comparison with open reduction method. Arch Orthop Trauma Surg 2003; 123(9):489–93.

97. Chen XZ, Liu CG, Chen Y, et al. Arthroscopy-assisted surgery for tibial plateau fractures. Arthroscopy 2015;31(1):143–53.

98. Saltzman CL, Salamon ML, Blanchard GM, et al. Epidemiology of ankle arthritis: report of a consecutive series of 639 patients from a tertiary orthopaedic center. Iowa Orthop J 2005;25:44–6.

99. Furman B, Olson S, Guilak F. The development of posttraumatic arthritis after articular fracture. J Orthop Trauma 2006;20(10):719–25.

100. Watson J, Moed B, Karges DE, et al. Pilon fractures: treatment protocol based on severity of the soft tissue. Clin Orthop Relat Res 2000;375: 78–90.

101. Tornetta P, Weiner L, Bergman M. Pilon fractures: treatment with combined internal and external fixation. J Orthop Trauma 1993;7:489–96.

102. Torino D, Mehta S. Fibular fixation in distal tibia fractures: reduction aid or nonunion generator? J Orthop Trauma 2016;30(Suppl 4):S22–5.

103. Lee YS, Chen SW, Chen SH, et al. Stabilisation of the fractured fibula plays an important role in the treatment of pilon fractures: a retrospective comparison of fibular fixation methods. Int Orthop 2009;33:695–9.

104. Kurylo J, Datta N, Iskander KN, et al. Does the fibula need to be fixed in complex pilon fractures? J Orthop Trauma 2015;9:424–7.

105. Bai J, Wang Y, Zhang P, et al. Efficacy and safety of 3D print-assisted surgery for the treatment of pilon fractures: a meta-analysis of randomized controlled trials. J Orthop Surg Res 2018;13(1):283.

Posttraumatic Arthritis After Intra-Articular Distal Femur and Proximal Tibia Fractures

Jacob T. Davis, MD[a,b,c,*], Matthew I. Rudloff, MD[a,b,c]

KEYWORDS

• Posttraumatic arthritis • Intra-articular fracture • Knee • Tibial plateau • Distal femur

---

KEY POINTS

• Posttraumatic arthritis (PTA) occurs after intra-articular fracture (IAF) about the knee and is a major cause of disability in young active patients.
• The goal of initial treatment after IAF is to limit future disability, primarily through restoration of the articular surface, joint stability, and limb alignment.
• Total knee arthroplasty (TKA) remains the mainstay of treatment for PTA and may be an option for initial treatment of IAF in some circumstances.

INTRODUCTION

Posttraumatic arthritis (PTA) is a form of joint degeneration that occurs after physical trauma to a synovial joint. Development of PTA is multi-factorial and results from mechanical damage at the time of trauma, inflammatory cell-mediated response, and abnormal articulation due to persistent malalignment or joint instability. PTA accounts for an estimated 12% of the cases of symptomatic arthritis of the lower extremities, affecting approximately 5.6 million individuals in the United States.[1] Patients present in a manner similar to primary osteoarthritis (OA); however, they have a history of an inciting traumatic event such as fracture. PTA is estimated to occur in approximately 23% to 36% of cases following intra-articular fracture (IAF) about the knee.[2–4] This incidence appears unchanged with time, despite advancements in fracture care.[5,6]

Most IAFs occur in patients younger than 45, and patients who develop PTA are on average 9 to 14 years younger than those with OA.[1] This makes the treatment of PTA difficult, as patients are often younger, more active, and have higher functional demands than those with OA. Most cases of degenerative arthritis of the knee in patients younger than 50 years are due to PTA.[7] Factors that have been shown to influence poor outcomes include severity of injury, articular incongruity or malalignment, associated soft tissue injury, and age at time of injury. Open anatomic reduction with internal fixation is the treatment of choice for articular fractures, although nonoperative management or primary arthroplasty may be considered in some. Conversion to total knee arthroplasty (TKA) is the mainstay of treatment for PTA, and results in significant improvements in function. Outcomes after reconstruction have historically been worse than for primary TKA for OA, including reoperation rates as high as

---

Disclosure Statement: Dr Rudloff receives Educational consulting from Smith and Nephew and Royalties from Elsevier.
[a] Department of Orthopaedic Surgery and Biomedical Engineering, University of Tennessee-Campbell Clinic, 1211 Union Avenue, Suite 520, Memphis, TN 38104, USA; [b] Regional One Health Medical Center, 877 Jefferson Avenue, Memphis, TN 38103, USA; [c] The Campbell Foundation, 1211 Union Avenue, Suite 500, Memphis, TN 38104, USA
* Corresponding author. The Campbell Foundation, 1211 Union Avenue, Suite 500, Memphis, TN 38104.
E-mail address: JTDavis52@gmail.com

21%.[8–10] However, recent advances in arthroplasty techniques have led to promising improvements in long-term survivorship and patient-reported functional outcomes.[11]

PATHOGENESIS

The pathogenesis of PTA is multifactorial but always follows a traumatic event. PTA of the knee is common following anterior cruciate ligament (ACL) and meniscal tears. A meta-analysis found that specified knee injuries (ligament injury, meniscus tear, or fracture) are associated with an increased risk of developing PTA, with an odds ratio of 5.95 (95% confidence interval 4.57–7.75).[12] The joint degeneration may result from damage at the time of trauma, such as IAF or cartilage injury, the resulting inflammatory cellular response, or abnormal articulation due to persistent malalignment or joint instability from ligamentous injury.[5] The likelihood of developing PTA is due to a combination of these factors and the sensitivity of a joint to resultant articular step-off is inversely proportional to the thickness of the articular cartilage.[13,14] It also has been postulated that the severity of the acute articular damage determines how well that cartilage tolerates long-term mechanical changes.[15]

The acute articular damage occurs at the time of traumatic injury and varies widely in severity from nondisplaced to highly comminuted fractures with impaction of the articular surface. The fracture severity is determined by the force imparted, the position of the extremity at the time of impact, and the quality of underlying bone. A low-energy mechanism in an elderly patient with poor bone quality will result in a more severe fracture pattern than in someone with more robust bone. It is logical that a nondisplaced fracture with little to no disruption of the articular cartilage is at low risk of development of PTA. However, if a simple fracture is associated with ligamentous injury that is not addressed, the chronic instability may lead to end-stage degeneration over the course of years. Conversely, a very comminuted fracture, such as a ballistic injury, would be at very high risk for rapid development of PTA.

Articular cartilage consists of mostly water and a solid matrix of collagen, proteoglycans, and chondrocytes. It is a unique structure that is strong against repetitive use but sensitive to direct force. Fractures involving the articular surface cause cartilage damage both mechanically and biologically. This cartilage damage also occurs along a timeline from immediately at the time of injury, through cytokine-mediated cell death, and finally to end-stage degenerative changes from chronic joint overload. Damage to the articular cartilage that occurs at the time of injury is due to mechanical force; this is one of the most important factors in the development of PTA.[16] The degree of fracture comminution, articular depression, ligamentous injury, and cartilage damage are dependent on the force applied, the position of the knee, and the strength of the underlying bone. Highly comminuted fracture lines may contain minute or nonreconstructable osteochondral fragments that, if small enough, are removed during surgery. Cartilaginous flaps or fragments may be fractured off as well leading to bare areas of exposed bone.

Not all damage is done at the time of injury, in the following days an inflammatory cascade, modulated by cytokines, proceeds to cause further cartilage damage. Following an IAF, synovial fluid has been shown to exhibit a proinflammatory cytokine mix similar to that of OA, which leads to cartilage extracellular matrix degradation.[17] Elevation of these cytokines, including interleukin (IL)-6, IL-8, and matrix metalloproteinases (MMPs) persists in synovial fluid even after bony union.[18] The role of cytokines in chondrocyte death is an emerging area of research. A 3-phase concept of tissue damage following articular injury has been proposed by Anderson and colleagues,[19] which includes an early phase of cell death/apoptosis (0–2 days), an intermediate phase of cytokine-mediated inflammation (3–9 days), and a late phase of chronic inflammation. The early phase includes chondrocyte necrosis, which been shown to be induced by a single rapid load and the extent is related to the amount of force applied.[20] Thus, the energy imparted onto the knee joint at the time of injury will determine the amount of chondrocyte death. Following this in the early phase is a rise in proinflammatory cytokines (IL-1β and IL-6) and factors such as caspases, which can induce chondrocyte apoptosis.[21] Caspases are enzymes that regulate apoptosis and studies have shown their increase following joint injury. It has been demonstrated in vitro that caspase inhibition can prevent chondrocyte apoptosis.[22] The second phase is induced by a surge in mediators of cartilage catabolism and is characterized by products of heme and cartilage breakdown.[23] The late phase is characterized by limited remodeling and progressive degeneration of articular cartilage.[21]

Chronic abnormal joint overload, be it from articular incongruity, instability, or malalignment, leads to continual degeneration. This loading affects the composition, structure, metabolic activity, and mechanical properties of articular cartilage leading to changes similar to OA.[24] The poor ability of cartilage, especially with preexisting arthritic changes, to tolerate this overload is likely why older patients have been found to do worse.

PREVENTION

As the development of PTA is a complex process, prevention of PTA requires a multifaceted approach. The balance of factors contributing to the development of PTA varies between joints and even in different areas within the same joint. Fracture about the tibial plateau seems to tolerate articular incongruities better than fractures of other joints; however, it appears that the knee is less tolerant to joint instability, removal of the meniscus, and coronal malalignment.[25] Although severity of the injury and the resulting damage done at that time cannot be undone, there are strategies to mitigate further damage. The primary strategy for fixation of displaced IAF focuses on anatomic reduction of the articular surface and stable internal fixation.[13] It is clear that restoration of alignment and stability are crucial as well. Future steps to mitigate damage done by inflammatory cytokines will be integral to the prevention of PTA.

One of the most important factors influencing the development of PTA may be unavoidable. It has been shown that the risk of PTA increases with age. Age has been shown to greatly affect the ability of chondrocytes to respond to anabolic stimuli; this has been linked to cell senescence.[26] A higher likelihood of preexisting arthritis and lower ability to heal leads older individuals significantly more at risk for the development of PTA. Clinical studies also have shown an increased incidence of PTA with increasing age.[7,27] Stevens and colleagues[28] showed that higher age at the time of injury was the most significant source of variation in outcome and increasing age at presentation lead to a trend toward worse functional outcome scores. In a review of 83 bicondylar tibial plateau fractures treated with medial and lateral plate fixation through 2 exposures, Barei and colleagues[29] showed that age was associated with worse scores on the Musculoskeletal Function Assessment.

There is conflicting evidence about the link between articular incongruity and the development of PTA in the knee. This link has clearly been established for fractures of the acetabulum, with residual displacement >2 mm being linked to poor outcomes.[30] It has also been shown for acetabular fractures that step displacement is tolerated less than gap displacement, with step displacement of 1 mm tolerated worse than gap displacement of 5 mm, with respect to the need for conversion to total hip arthroplasty.[31] This difference in articular incongruity between the hip and the knee is likely due to the presence of the meniscus and larger joint surface area. Although the link between reduction and PTA is less clear for fractures of the tibial plateau, some investigators have found an association whereas others have not.[25]

Historical studies have found that residual articular incongruity up to 10 mm is well tolerated and does not compromise functional outcomes.[2,27,32–38] These studies have been criticized for outdated treatment strategies and inconsistent outcome measures; however, there are historical articles that do conclude that adequacy of reduction is important in obtaining satisfactory results. In 1984, Blokker and colleagues[39] asserted that the single most influential factor in predicting outcome was the adequacy of reduction. This should be considered in context, as the threshold of articular step-off >5 mm was associated with unsatisfactory results and it was acknowledged that step-off <5 mm did not preclude a good result. More recently, a study by Barei and colleagues[29] demonstrated better patient-reported functional outcomes when a satisfactory articular reduction was achieved. This satisfactory articular reduction of ≤2 mm step-off or gap was achieved in only 55% of their patients. In 2017, Singleton and colleagues[40] found that larger residual joint depression (>2.5 mm) results in a greater loss of motion and worse patient-reported outcome scores. In a review article about articular step-off, Giannoudis and colleagues[25] state that for fractures of the tibial plateau, "most authors agree that the acceptable range of intra-articular step-off is in the range of 2 to 10 mm." In a publication based on an American Orthopedic Association symposium, Marsh and colleagues[16] assert that, "there is little rationale, on the basis of the evidence available in the literature, for the assertion that accurate articular reduction of tibial plateau fracture, particularly to tolerances of <2 mm, is critical to the attainment of a good clinical outcome."

Animal studies have demonstrated that step offs greater than the average thickness of the articular cartilage cannot successfully remodel, but those incongruities up to the size of the depth of cartilage have the ability to restore a near normal surface.[25] This applies to IAF of both the distal femur and proximal tibia. It has been shown that the mean cartilage thickness of the knee is significantly greater than that of the hip and ankle. The average thickness of the cartilage on the femoral condyles is 1.65 to 2.65 mm. The area of the tibia not covered by meniscus that is in direct contact with the femoral condyle has an average cartilage thickness of 2.07 to 2.98 mm.[41] Although effort should be made to restore articular congruity to the best of the surgeon's abilities, the benefits of a reduction to narrower tolerances than the articular cartilage should be weighed against the risks associated with the insult of open reduction.[16]

Stability and alignment likely play larger roles than articular congruity in the prevention of PTA of the knee.[5] Accepted standards for satisfactory alignment of the distal femur is 6° ± 5° of valgus and of the proximal tibia is 3° ± 5° of varus in the coronal plane and 9° ± 5° of posterior slope in the sagittal plane.[29] In a study of 131 tibial plateau fractures, Honkonen[36] found that clinical function was worse with any residual varus angulation but valgus angulation was well tolerated up to 5°. Rasmussen[42] reported similar findings, with OA developing in 19 (13%) of 146 patients with valgus angulation less than 10° and 6 (54.5%) of 11 patients with valgus angulation greater than 10°.

The stability of the tibiofemoral articulation results from a complex interaction of static anatomic structures and dynamic physiologic mechanisms.[43] Joint laxity is an objective finding of excessive joint movement; this is one factor that contributes to instability, which is a subjective sensation of buckling or giving way during functional activities.[44] The link between joint stability and the development of PTA has been well established, even in the absence of fracture. In a review of knee dislocations, Moatshe and colleagues[45] found that 27 (42%) of 65 of surgically treated knee dislocations developed OA at a minimum of 10-year follow-up. Older age (>30 years) at time of knee dislocation was associated with development of OA. In the previously mentioned review by Honkonen,[36] he also concluded that 70% of knees with moderate to severe instability had unacceptable functional outcomes. In a series of tibial plateau fractures Lansinger and colleagues[34] noted that unstable fracture with residual depression of more than 10 mm had inferior results. They concluded that the determination of operative management should be based on stability of the knee and not radiographic appearance. Delamarter and colleagues[46] found poor results in 10 of 12 patients with 10° or more of residual laxity, these were in 5 unrepaired medial collateral ligaments, 2 unrepaired lateral collateral ligaments, and 3 cruciate ligament injuries.

Other factors clearly linked to the development of PTA are meniscectomy and postoperative infection. Meniscectomy was historically performed with the assumption that it had little effect on joint function; however, it has been conclusively shown that complete meniscectomy results in high rates of degenerative arthritis, even without IAF.[47,48] Honkonen[36] found that OA developed in 20 (74%) of 27 knees following meniscectomy and in 18 (36.7%) of 49 knees that did not undergo meniscectomy. It is currently recommended to assess the condition of the meniscus intraoperatively and repair the meniscus as indicated.[49]

Currently no treatment strategies are widely used to prevent cartilage damage from the inflammatory cascade. Biological treatments targeting cytokine mitigation to prevent inflammatory-mediated cartilage damage represent an exciting future direction for prevention of PTA. As such, the mainstay of prevention of PTA remains the restoration of the mechanical aspects of the knee's articulation.

EVALUATION

Evaluation of the initial injury is routinely with standard radiograph and may include a computed tomography (CT) scan to assess the extent of articular involvement. This can demonstrate markers of poor outcome, such as comminution, impaction, and extensive articular involvement. Occasionally MRI is warranted to evaluate the extent of soft tissue injury. MRI is useful to show the presence and degree of ligamentous, meniscal, or cartilage injury.

Tibial plateau fractures are routinely classified based on the classic description by Schatzker and colleagues.[50] Although they can also be classified based on the AO Foundation/Orthopaedic Trauma Association (AO/OTA) classification system as 41B and 41C fractures. Fractures of the distal femur do not have classic fracture patterns or widely used classification systems. They are more commonly classified based on descriptive terms, such as having simple or comminuted involvement of the metaphysis with simple or complex extension to the articular surface. The AO/OTA fracture classification group 33 is used for these fractures.

The question of when MRI is indicated in tibial plateau fractures remains unanswered. The amount of lateral joint depression has been associated with rate of lateral meniscal tear, with an odds ratio of 1.36.[49] In a prospective diagnostic study of 102 patients, Chang and colleagues[51] used arthroscopy after internal fixation of tibial plateau fractures and found meniscal injury in 54 (52.9%) patients and cruciate ligament injury in 23 (22.5%) patients. There was a greater risk of lateral meniscus injury in patients with more than 6.3 mm of lateral joint depression and a greater risk of ACL injury with greater than 5.7 mm of joint widening, indicating that these may help predict the risk of soft tissue injury. In a review of 103 MRIs on consecutive acute tibial plateau fractures Gardner and colleagues[52] found a high incidence of associated soft tissue injuries, including 91% lateral meniscal tear, 44% medial meniscal tear, 77% ligamentous tear, and 68% had tears of posterior lateral corner structures. These investigators admit that the clinical importance of injury to these structures is unknown. In a later article from the same academic center, Warner and colleagues[53] found that untreated medial meniscus tears and complete medial collateral ligament ruptures did not significantly affect clinical outcomes. In their series of 82 operatively treated tibial plateau fractures followed for a minimum of 12 months, 8 (9.8%) were found to have ACL tears on MRI, only 1 of which went onto delayed reconstruction. These studies call into question the clinical necessity of routine MRI and may indicate that intraoperative assessment of the meniscus during fixation of displaced tibial plateau fractures and physical examination of ligamentous stability after fixation with consideration for repair of unstable structures may be adequate for most fractures. The decision to obtain a preoperative MRI should remain at the discretion of the treating surgeon.

Several techniques exist to evaluate the adequacy of the articular reduction after fixation of IAF. Direct visualization of the articular surface is routinely afforded in the knee, either through a parapatellar capsulotomy for the distal femur or through a sub-meniscal arthrotomy for the tibial plateau. Intraoperative fluoroscopy, which though limited, allows for visualization of articular congruity and alignment. A recent cadaver study by Haller and colleagues[54] showed that anteroposterior and lateral fluoroscopy was only able to detect, with high interobserver agreement, 2 mm and 5 mm step-off. Their conclusion is that visualization of the articular surface is necessary to ensure anatomic reduction. Intraoperative 3-dimensional (3D) imaging is an emerging technique that can improve visualization of articular reduction. A cadaver study evaluating the ability to detect 1 mm and 2 mm of joint line step-off compared conventional fluoroscopy, CT scan, and intraoperative 3D fluoroscopy showed improved visualization

with 3D fluoroscopy over conventional fluoroscopy.[55] Postoperative radiography or CT can be used to ensure extra-articular placement of implants and assess the adequacy of articular reduction, as well as alignment of the mechanical axis.

PTA is most commonly graded using standardized scoring systems for OA, such as the Kellgran-Lawrence or International Knee Documentation Committee grading systems. These classifications are based on the presence or absence of osteophytes, joint space narrowing, subchondral cystic changes, and sclerosis or deformity of the bone ends. Both systems have been validated with respect to intraobserver and interobserver reliability and have been shown to have high diagnostic accuracy, especially when using Rosenberg radiographs (45° flexion weightbearing posteroanterior radiograph).[56] It should be noted that radiographic evidence of OA does not correlate with symptoms or poor function.[13]

Evaluation of radiographic degenerative changes may be limited by fixation implants about the knee. Occasionally implants are removed before evaluation for reconstruction; this is usually at the discretion of the treating surgeons or based on patient preference. If malunion is present, it is helpful to measure the degree of deformity in the sagittal and coronal plane, as significant deformity may preclude routine reconstructive options for PTA. It may be necessary to perform an osteotomy of the distal femur or proximal tibia to restore anatomic alignment prior or in conjunction TKA.

MANAGEMENT AND OUTCOMES: FIXATION

The mainstay of treatment of displaced IAF of the knee joint is an open approach for direct reduction with the goal of anatomic alignment of the articular surface and mechanical axis of the limb. Soft tissue repairs also may be indicated at the time of surgery, including meniscal repair or ligament reconstruction (Box 1).

Treatment of fractures of the distal femur is predominantly surgical with nonsurgical management reserved for truly nondisplaced fractures and patients whose medical problems preclude safe surgical intervention, as nonsurgical management is associated with worse clinical outcomes.[57,58] The hallmark of treatment of IAF of the distal femur is open reduction of the articular surface with indirect reduction of the metaphysis, if comminution is present. The choice of implant, between retrograde nail and

---

Box 1
Goals of treatment of intra-articular fracture of the knee

Anatomic articular surface

Restoration of condylar width

Mechanical axis alignment

Joint stability

Repair of soft tissues

---

plate and screw fixation, is determined by the fracture pattern and the preference of the treating surgeon. Some surgeons prefer retrograde intramedullary nail fixation of fractures with simple intra-articular splits (AO/OTA 33C1 and C2), with direct reduction and lag screw fixation of the articular surface. This has shown to lead to a low rates of nonunion, malunion, and subsequent bone grafting.[59] Anatomic distal femur plates are still preferred by some, especially for comminuted IAF of the distal femur (AO/OTA 33C3), although rate of nonunion remains a worry, especially with open and high-energy fracture, with rates of 18% to 35% previously reported.[60,61] However, recent study by Wenger and Andersson[62] of 191 fractures treated at a nontertiary referral center found that 8 (4%) patients developed nonunion. They postulated that high rates previously were due to a predominance of literature coming from tertiary referral centers with a high percentage of high-energy and open fracture (Fig. 1).

Outcomes after open reduction internal fixation (ORIF) of IAF of the distal femur are good with a low rate of subsequent TKA. In a report of 22 distal femur fractures, Thomson and colleagues[59] found that 12 (54.5%) had significant degenerative changes; however, none had undergone TKA. Of 30 distal femur fractures available for long-term follow-up, Rademakers and colleagues[3] found moderate to severe OA developed in 11 (36.7%) patients. Of patients who had developed arthritis, 8 (72%) had good to excellent Neer scores.

Isolated condylar fractures that occur in the coronal plane are injuries that were originally described in 1904 by Hoffa. These fractures may be missed on routine radiography, and missed injuries and nonoperative treatment have been associated with a high rate of displacement. ORIF is recommended, which results in good outcomes.[63] Hoffa fractures frequently occur in association with high-energy distal femur fractures, with rates as high as 38%, and more often involve the lateral

condyle. Preoperative CT scan is recommended to assess for this fracture pattern.[64] Fixation of these fractures with small fragment lag screws has shown to be adequate with low rates of displacement. In a review of 56 coronal plane fractures associated with intercondylar distal femur fractures, Telleria and colleagues[65] found only 1 (1.8%) went on to avascular necrosis.

Nonoperative management of tibial plateau fractures is more common than for distal femur fractures. Acceptable functional outcomes can be achieved with nonsurgical management in fractures with minimal displacement or depression that are stable to varus and valgus. It is also recommended in nonambulatory or medically unstable patients.

Due to unfavorable results with TKA after ORIF of tibial plateau fractures, some investigators suggest initial nonoperative treatment of IAF in the elderly or those with preexisting arthritis with delayed TKA as indicated, although nonoperative management is limited to those fractures with reasonable alignment, which would facilitate a straightforward TKA. In fractures with significant displacement or altered alignment, a limited fixation procedure can be used to reconstitute bone stock for a delayed total knee procedure. It is helpful in this circumstance to be mindful of future arthroplasty approaches and consider a more anterior midline approach, as described by Starr and colleagues.[66,67]

Honkonen[36] in 1994 laid out indications for surgical treatment of proximal tibia fractures, including valgus angulation greater than 5°, step-off >3 mm, widening >5 mm, any displaced fracture of the medial plateau, and bicondylar fractures (except those with nondisplaced medial plateau with lateral fractures meeting nonoperative criteria) (Box 2). He also concluded that all collateral ligament damage leading to instability in extension after fixation and all ACL avulsions leading to instability should be repaired.[36] Operative fixation proceeds with an open approach, as dictated by the fracture pattern. This can be an anterolateral or posteromedial approach or both. Fixation can be achieved by subchondral lag screws along the joint followed by buttress plate fixation for partial articular injuries. For bicondylar tibial plateau fractures, medial and lateral small fragment plates or a lateral-based large fragment plate may be used for fixation.[29]

For fracture with simple intra-articular extension but complex metaphyseal involvement, an intramedullary nail is also an option. Mini fragment plates and screws can be used as adjuncts

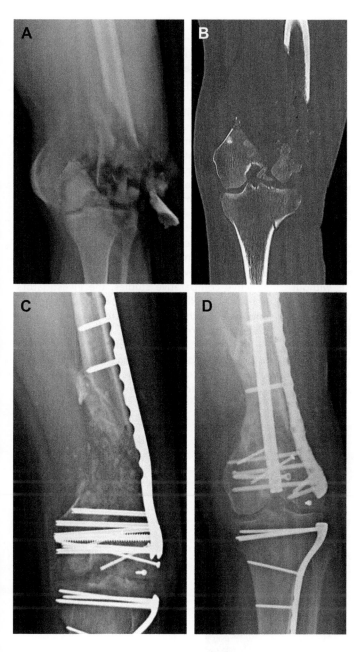

Fig. 1. (A, B) Preoperative radiograph and coronal CT images demonstrating highly comminuted and open distal femur and tibial plateau fractures. (C) A follow-up radiograph 4 months after injury. The patient underwent interval bone graft procedure; however, developed implant failure requiring revision. (D) A follow-up radiograph 16 months after injury demonstrating solid bony union with preservation of joint space.

in comminuted fractures or to hold provisional reductions in combination with more stable implants. Limited internal fixation with external fixation is another technique recommended by some investigators. External fixation can be accomplished with a circular external fixator or a temporary knee spanning uniplanar external fixator.[2]

Some fracture patterns are more predictive of poor outcomes than others. High-energy and bicondylar plateaus have been shown to have worse results.[4] The hyperextension pattern of

tibial plateau fracture has been shown to be a predictor of poor outcome (Fig. 2). Egol and colleagues[68] showed that 5 (33.3%) of 15 patients with hyperextension pattern tibial plateau fractures went onto PTA, compared with 7 (10.1%) of 69 patients with nonhyperextension bicondylar fractures.

Historical meniscectomy had been a common treatment for meniscal tears in association with open treatment of tibial plateau fractures; this practice has been abandoned due to poor outcomes. In a report of 101 acute tibial plateau fractures Forman and colleagues[49] suggest that acute repair of the meniscus in conjunction with open treatment of the fracture can yield functional outcomes similar to patients without meniscal tears.

Another technique that has been proposed for treatment of tibial plateau fractures is arthroscopic-assisted reduction with internal fixation (ARIF). Originally described in 1985 by Caspari and colleagues[69] and Jennings,[70] it has in limited case series shown advantages by allowing direct visualization and accurate diagnosis and treatment of associated intra-articular soft tissue injuries. A reported risk of this technique includes extravasation of arthroscopy fluid leading to compartment syndrome of the leg or thigh.[71] As this is a devastating consequence, it should be monitored for and it is recommended by most articles to use gravity instead of pump inflow. A recent review article out of China included 19 studies with 609 patients, and compartment syndrome was reported in only 1 case. Associated intra-articular soft tissue injuries were common, including 42.2% meniscal injuries and 21.3% ACL injuries. This technique is mostly used for low-energy, Schatzker type II and III, injuries and especially those with concomitant intra-articular injuries. Although limited to a review of case series and 2 retrospective comparative studies, the investigators concluded ARIF to be a "reliable, effective, and safe method for the treatment of tibial plateau fractures."[72]

In elderly patients without preexisting arthritis, poor bone quality may compromise stable internal fixation. A combination plate-and-nail construct for distal femur and proximal tibia

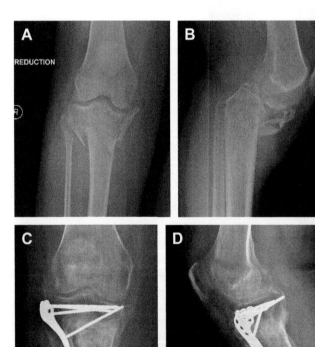

Fig. 2. (*A*, *B*) Preoperative radiographs demonstrating extension-type tibial plateau fracture with considerable anterior cortical comminution. (*C*, *D*) Radiographs 5 months after fixation demonstrate varus collapse but maintenance of posterior slope of the proximal tibia.

fractures in these patients has been described to facilitate early weightbearing.[73] There are reports in the literature of allowing full weightbearing for distal femur fractures in geriatric patients with no increased rate of complications.[74] However, this is primarily for extraarticular fractures, although in this patient population the risk of intra-articular displacement may be of lower concern than mobilization.

MANAGEMENT AND OUTCOMES: PRIMARY ARTHROPLASTY

One option for treatment of distal femur fractures in the geriatric population is primary TKA with a distal femoral replacement (DFR) or hinged prosthesis (**Fig. 3**). In a review of 24 DFRs for distal femur fracture with mean follow-up of 11 months, Rosen and Strauss[75] reported no major complications and 17 (71%) had returned to their preoperative level of ambulation. Appleton and colleagues[76] described using a hinged TKA in 52 elderly patients with distal femur fractures; the 1-year mortality was 41%, but those who survived returned to their preinjury level of function. In a study by Bettin and colleagues,[77] 18 patients

with average age of 77 years were treated with cemented, modular DFR. They reported 2 (11.1%) implant-related complications, 1 deep infection, and 1 periprosthetic fracture. In their cohort, 4 were open fractures initially treated with debridement and irrigation and staged conversion to DFR, none of which became infected. At an average of 2-year follow-up, there was no evidence of aseptic loosening.

Primary arthroplasty for tibial plateau fractures is less commonly reported in the literature, this is likely because there are major concerns with this technique, including tibial component subsidence and extensor mechanism integrity. Occasionally a combination of ORIF and arthroplasty with constrained components is required, as described by Weinlein and colleagues.[78] An anterior-based approach is performed and provisional fixation with screws or a plate is obtained being mindful to avoid the intramedullary canal to allow for broaching of the tibial canal. The proximal tibial cut is then performed and a stemmed tibial component is inserted, with metaphyseal sleeve or impaction grafting as indicated. In a recent series of 30 patients undergoing acute TKA for

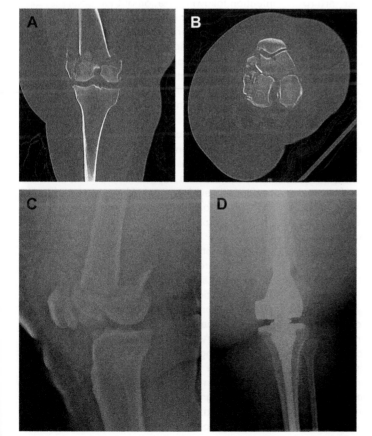

Fig. 3. (*A, B*) Coronal and axial CT images demonstrating a very distal and highly comminuted distal femur fracture in a morbidly obese patient. (*C*) A lateral radiograph that demonstrates the displacement. The injury was deemed to not be reconstructible and (*D*) distal femur replacement was performed.

tibial fracture, Haufe and colleagues[79] reported good functional outcomes with mean follow-up of 27 months. However, there were 7 (23.3%) reoperations for complications and 2 (6.7%) deaths attributed to reoperation.

DECISION MAKING BETWEEN OPEN REDUCTION INTERNAL FIXATION AND TOTAL KNEE ARTHROPLASTY

The field of orthopedics has moved heavily toward replacement for fractures about the shoulder, elbow, and hip. However, there is limited literature on acute replacement for fractures about the knee despite excellent options for knee arthroplasty. Geriatric patients with distal femur fractures are similar in many ways to those with proximal femur fractures.[74,80,81] However, less attention is given to early surgery, constructs that allow early weightbearing, and perioperative management in these patients in comparison with patients with fractures of the proximal femur. With superior results following total hip arthroplasty for displaced femoral neck fractures, it would follow that patients would mobilize sooner and may return to a higher level of independence after TKA for distal femur fracture.[78] Treatment, whether arthroplasty or fixation, of geriatric distal femur and proximal tibia fractures should be performed in a timely fashion and in a manner allowing early weightbearing if feasible. Constructs such as the combination of a plate and intramedullary nail can offer early weightbearing in extra-articular fractures, negating the advantage of arthroplasty. This may be applicable to fracture with a simple intra-articular split.

Acute TKA for IAF about the knee should be considered in older patients, those with preexisting symptomatic arthritis, severe osteoporosis precluding stable fixation, and articular fractures considered nonreconstructible. It also should be considered that immediate weightbearing after internal fixation of osteoporotic fractures with significant comminution and intra-articular extension may lead to early failure, and arthroplasty would have a distinct advantage in this situation.[78]

Two studies compare arthroplasty with ORIF for distal femur fractures, one concluded that TKA had better range of motion and more return to independent ambulation.[82] The other found no difference in reoperation or deep infection, but ORIF had an 18% rate of nonunion and trended toward higher rate of wheelchair dependency.[83] These studies are limited by small sample size and short-term follow-up; it remains up to the treating surgeon and the patient to decide the best way to proceed with regard to fixation or replacement.

MANAGEMENT AND OUTCOMES: DELAYED RECONSTRUCTION

Overall the rate of tibial plateau fractures leading to end-stage PTA requiring TKA is low. Wasserstein and colleagues[84] found 7.3% incidence of TKA at 10 years after operatively treated tibial plateau fracture. This was based on a series of 8426 patients compared with 33,698 matched controls. The need for TKA was associated with increasing age, severity of fracture (bicondylar), and soft tissue injury, including meniscal tear. The incidence of TKA at 10 years after bicondylar tibial plateau fracture was 11%. Other series have reported risk factors to also include limb malalignment[4] (Fig. 4).

TKA for posttraumatic arthritis leads to significant improvements in functional outcomes, but has historically worse outcomes than TKA for primary OA.[85] In 2001, a failure rate of 33% was reported in 15 patients undergoing TKA for PTA, 2 for patellar tendon disruption and 3 for infection,[9] especially in those with previous infection following fixation of their tibial plateau, with up to 4.1 times high reoperation rates than those with no prior infection.[86] In a review article Saleh and colleagues[87] found that TKA for PTA results in improved pain, range of motion, and functional outcomes scores; however, it is associated with higher rates of complications, including infection, stiffness, wound complications, extensor tendon rupture, and polyethylene wear. Reported rates of revision in 9 studies that they included were 3% to 18%. Survivorship in various studies has been reported at 79% to 90% with various end points; there is conflicting evidence whether survivorship is lower than for TKA for OA. The overwhelming majority of complications were noted in the first 2 years.

Arthroplasty following distal femur fracture is similarly more complicated, due to scarring, nonunion, malunion, or infection; however, significant function improvement can be obtained with TKA after distal femur fracture. Papadopoulos and colleagues[88] reported on 48 cemented condylar TKAs for PTA after distal femur fracture, including 3 nonunions and 21 severe malunions. Knee range of motion as well as knee society pain and functional scores were improved significantly. However, deep infection was noted in 3 (6.2%), aseptic loosening in 2 (4.2%), arthrodesis in 1 (2.1%), and amputation

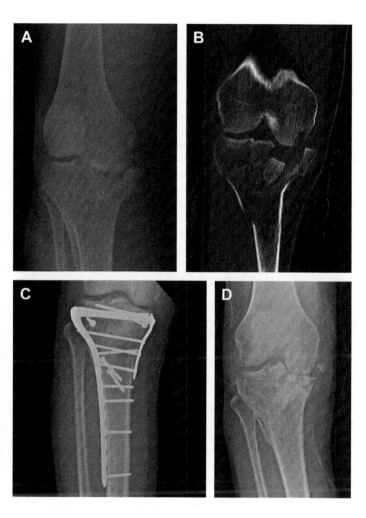

Fig. 4. (A) Medially depressed bicondylar tibial plateau fracture. (B) An isolated coronal CT view demonstrates high degree of comminution and associated distal femur fracture. (C) A postoperative radiograph demonstrates restoration of the articular surface but residual varus alignment. (D) Follow-up radiograph less than 6 months after surgery which demonstrates the development of significant PTA; the patient underwent removal of implants in preparation for staged TKA reconstruction.

in 1 (2.1%). In this cohort, good to excellent results were obtained in only 52% of patients.[88]

Recent studies have demonstrated more positive outcomes; this is reportedly due to modern techniques and implants. A report on 25 patients undergoing TKA for PTA using metaphyseal sleeves with semiconstrained rotating platform demonstrated good results with 100% survivorship at mean follow-up of 79 months.[89] Abdel and colleagues[90] reported on 62 patients who underwent TKA after a prior tibial plateau fracture and found 96% 15-year survivorship free from aseptic loosening. However, they reported complications in 21 (34%), more than 90% occurring less than 2 years after the TKA, and the survivorship at 15 years free from any revision was only 82%. They concluded that although patients undergoing TKA after tibial plateau fractures have increased rates of complications, survivorship is similar to that of TKA for OA if early complications can be avoided. Retrospectively reviewing a single institutions registry, 75 patients undergoing TKA for PTA were matched 5:1 to patients with OA. They found no difference in patient-reported outcomes measures or rate of revision between the 2 groups. Revision was required in 3% of patients with OA and 4% for patients with PTA; however, they excluded patients younger than 60 years and those with open fractures, and the mean follow-up was 7.5 years.[11]

FUTURE DIRECTIONS

The inflammatory cascade set off by the acute injury is one of the main targets of future research. Cytokine mitigation in the early period may improve clinical outcomes. Research is ongoing to develop strategies to decrease the inflammatory response to injury to minimize chondrocyte apoptosis, limit cartilage matrix degradation, and enhance matrix production. Treatments aimed against the early phase would need to be administered promptly after injury, and may be an intra-articular injection of an anti-inflammatory, particularly targeting caspases and IL-1. Therapies targeting the second and third phases of tissue damage would target preventing matrix degradation and promoting matrix regeneration.[21]

Research is under way to better understand these factors, which may lead to novel treatment strategies, including therapeutic targets to inhibit caspases. In an impact test of freshly harvested human ankle cartilage, an amphipathic nonionic surfactant poloxamer P188 was shown to prevent cell death and inhibit the spread of chondrocyte apoptosis into non-impacted areas. P188 exerts these positive effects by stabilizing the cell membrane to prevent the propagation of signaling pathways involved in impact-related damage. Specifically, P188 inhibits apoptosis-related activation of glycogen synthase kinase-3 (GSK3) and inflammation-related IL-6 signaling.[91] Although biological treatments will not replace the need for surgical management of IAF, in the future they may serve as vital adjuncts in the prevention of PTA.[21]

A recent animal study using sclerostin transgenic and knockout mice demonstrated mice given an intra-articular injection of sclerostin immediately post injury showed decreased proteolytic enzyme, including MMP, activity and prevents cartilage degradation.[92] Due to the elevated inflammatory cytokine mix, there are some who recommend consideration of early evacuation of the hemarthrosis associated with IAF.[23]

Genetic factors have been shown to contribute greatly to the susceptibility to OA. Specifically, single nucleotide polymorphisms have been found that reduce the expression of genes involved in the development of cartilage. These include growth differentiation factor-5, estrogen receptor-α, and calmodulin-1.[93] These, and possibly other, genetic risk factors may put affected patients at risk for development of PTA. Identification of genetic factors in the injury period may guide treatment, such as indicating arthroplasty over fixation in susceptible individuals.

One emerging technique for treatment of tibial plateau fractures is balloon tibioplasty for reduction of depressed segments of the articular surface. This uses a kyphoplasty balloon percutaneously placed beneath the area of depression, it is then inflated to provide an even reduction force, reduction is confirmed with fluoroscopy or arthroscopy, and this cavity is then filled with calcium phosphate bone cement. This may be a useful tool to facilitate accurate articular reduction.[94]

SUMMARY

PTA after IAF of the distal femur or proximal tibia results from damage to the articular surface from multiple factors. PTA occurs somewhat frequently and is a major cause of knee OA in young to middle-aged patients, leading to significant morbidity and loss of function. Initial treatment of these fractures aims to minimize long-term disability by restoring a stable, well-aligned, and anatomic articulation between the femur and the tibia. This is routinely accomplished with operative fixation. Primary arthroplasty is also an option in elderly patients and may allow early weightbearing, which benefits mobility in these fragile patients. Factors that determine outcomes after fixation and primary arthroplasty remain unclear and have yet to be thoroughly studied. This decision is usually based on the treating surgeon's impression of the fracture and patient factors, including age, functional level, and preexisting arthritis. Reconstructive options for PTA routinely include TKA, although it is complicated by the prior injury and comes at increased risks over primary TKA for OA. Advancements in TKA implants and techniques may narrow this disparity in functional outcomes in the future; however, reconstruction of PTA will remain a challenge. Further study into mitigating chondrocyte death, including cytokine modulation, may decrease the rate of PTA in the future.

REFERENCES

1. Brown TD, Johnston RC, Saltzman CL, et al. Post-traumatic osteoarthritis: a first estimate of incidence, prevalence, and burden of disease. J Orthop Trauma 2006;20(10):739–44.
2. Weigel DP, Marsh JL. High-energy fractures of the tibial plateau. Knee function after longer follow-up. J Bone Joint Surg Am 2002;84-A(9):1541–51.
3. Rademakers MV, Kerkhoffs GM, Sierevelt IN, et al. Intra-articular fractures of the distal femur: a long-term follow-up study of surgically treated patients. J Orthop Trauma 2004;18(4):213–9.
4. Rademakers MV, Kerkhoffs GM, Sierevelt IN, et al. Operative treatment of 109 tibial plateau fractures: five- to 27-year follow-up results. J Orthop Trauma 2007;21(1):5–10.
5. Schenker ML, Mauck RL, Ahn J, et al. Pathogenesis and prevention of posttraumatic osteoarthritis after

intra-articular fracture. J Am Acad Orthop Surg 2014;22(1):20–8.

6. Aurich M, Koenig V, Hofmann G. Comminuted intraarticular fractures of the tibial plateau lead to posttraumatic osteoarthritis of the knee: current treatment review. Asian J Surg 2018;41(2):99–105.

7. Honkonen SE. Degenerative arthritis after tibial plateau fractures. J Orthop Trauma 1995;9(4):273–7.

8. Scott CE, Davidson E, MacDonald DJ, et al. Total knee arthroplasty following tibial plateau fracture: a matched cohort study. Bone Joint J 2015;97-B(4):532–8.

9. Saleh KJ, Sherman P, Katkin P, et al. Total knee arthroplasty after open reduction and internal fixation of fractures of the tibial plateau: a minimum five-year follow-up study. J Bone Joint Surg Am 2001;83-A(8):1144–8.

10. Weiss NG, Parvizi J, Trousdale RT, et al. Total knee arthroplasty in patients with a prior fracture of the tibial plateau. J Bone Joint Surg Am 2003;85-A(2):218–21.

11. Khoshbin A, Stavrakis A, Sharma A, et al. Patient-reported outcome measures of total knee arthroplasties for post-traumatic arthritis versus osteoarthritis: a short-term (5- to 10-year) retrospective matched cohort study. J Arthroplasty 2019;34(5):872–6.e1.

12. Muthuri SG, McWilliams DF, Doherty M, et al. History of knee injuries and knee osteoarthritis: a meta-analysis of observational studies. Osteoarthritis Cartilage 2011;19(11):1286–93.

13. Dirschl DR, Marsh JL, Buckwalter JA, et al. Articular fractures. J Am Acad Orthop Surg 2004;12(6):416–23.

14. Lefkoe TP, Walsh WR, Anastasatos J, et al. Remodeling of articular step-offs. Is osteoarthrosis dependent on defect size? Clin Orthop Relat Res 1995;(314):253–65.

15. McKinley TO, Borrelli J Jr, D'Lima DD, et al. Basic science of intra-articular fractures and posttraumatic osteoarthritis. J Orthop Trauma 2010;24(9):567–70.

16. Marsh JL, Buckwalter J, Gelberman R, et al. Articular fractures: does an anatomic reduction really change the result? J Bone Joint Surg Am 2002;84-A(7):1259–71.

17. Adams SB, Setton LA, Bell RD, et al. Inflammatory cytokines and matrix metalloproteinases in the synovial fluid after intra-articular ankle fracture. Foot Ankle Int 2015;36(11):1264–71.

18. Adams SB, Leimer EM, Setton LA, et al. Inflammatory microenvironment persists after bone healing in intra-articular ankle fractures. Foot Ankle Int 2017;38(5):479–84.

19. Anderson DD, Chubinskaya S, Guilak F, et al. Post-traumatic osteoarthritis: improved understanding and opportunities for early intervention. J Orthop Res 2011;29(6):802–9.

20. Borrelli J Jr, Tinsley K, Ricci WM, et al. Induction of chondrocyte apoptosis following impact load. J Orthop Trauma 2003;17(9):635–41.

21. Olson SA, Horne P, Furman B, et al. The role of cytokines in posttraumatic arthritis. J Am Acad Orthop Surg 2014;22(1):29–37.

22. D'Lima DD, Hashimoto S, Chen PC, et al. Prevention of chondrocyte apoptosis. J Bone Joint Surg Am 2001;83-A:25–6. Suppl 2(Pt 1).

23. Adams SB, Reilly RM, Huebner JL, et al. Time-dependent effects on synovial fluid composition during the acute phase of human intra-articular ankle fracture. Foot Ankle Int 2017;38(10):1055–63.

24. Furman BD, Olson SA, Guilak F. The development of posttraumatic arthritis after articular fracture. J Orthop Trauma 2006;20(10):719–25.

25. Giannoudis PV, Tzioupis C, Papathanassopoulos A, et al. Articular step-off and risk of post-traumatic osteoarthritis. Evidence today. Injury 2010;41(10):986–95.

26. Martin JA, Buckwalter JA. Roles of articular cartilage aging and chondrocyte senescence in the pathogenesis of osteoarthritis. Iowa Orthop J 2001;21:1–7.

27. Volpin G, Dowd GS, Stein H, et al. Degenerative arthritis after intra-articular fractures of the knee. Long-term results. J Bone Joint Surg Br 1990;72(4):634–8.

28. Stevens DG, Beharry R, McKee MD, et al. The long-term functional outcome of operatively treated tibial plateau fractures. J Orthop Trauma 2001;15(5):312–20.

29. Barei DP, Nork SE, Mills WJ, et al. Functional outcomes of severe bicondylar tibial plateau fractures treated with dual incisions and medial and lateral plates. J Bone Joint Surg Am 2006;88(8):1713–21.

30. Matta JM. Fractures of the acetabulum: accuracy of reduction and clinical results in patients managed operatively within three weeks after the injury. J Bone Joint Surg Am 1996;78(11):1632–45.

31. Verbeek DO, van der List JP, Tissue CM, et al. Predictors for long-term hip survivorship following acetabular fracture surgery: importance of gap compared with step displacement. J Bone Joint Surg Am 2018;100(11):922–9.

32. Lucht U, Pilgaard S. Fractures of the tibial condyles. Acta Orthop Scand 1971;42(4):366–76.

33. Rasmussen PS. Tibial condylar fractures as a cause of degenerative arthritis. Acta Orthop Scand 1972;43(6):566–75.

34. Lansinger O, Bergman B, Korner L, et al. Tibial condylar fractures. A twenty-year follow-up. J Bone Joint Surg Am 1986;68(1):13–9.

35. Duwelius PJ, Connolly JF. Closed reduction of tibial plateau fractures. A comparison of functional and roentgenographic end results. Clin Orthop Relat Res 1988;230:116–26.

36. Honkonen SE. Indications for surgical treatment of tibial condyle fractures. Clin Orthop Relat Res 1994;(302):199–205.

37. Koval KJ, Sanders R, Borrelli J, et al. Indirect reduction and percutaneous screw fixation of displaced tibial plateau fractures. J Orthop Trauma 1992; 6(3):340–6.

38. Waddell JP, Johnston DW, Neidre A. Fractures of the tibial plateau: a review of ninety-five patients and comparison of treatment methods. J Trauma 1981;21(5):376–81.

39. Blokker CP, Rorabeck CH, Bourne RB. Tibial plateau fractures. An analysis of the results of treatment in 60 patients. Clin Orthop Relat Res 1984;(182):193–9.

40. Singleton N, Sahakian V, Muir D. Outcome after tibial plateau fracture: how important is restoration of articular congruity? J Orthop Trauma 2017;31(3): 158–63.

41. Shepherd DE, Seedhom BB. Thickness of human articular cartilage in joints of the lower limb. Ann Rheum Dis 1999;58(1):27–34.

42. Rasmussen PS. Tibial condylar fractures. Impairment of knee joint stability as an indication for surgical treatment. J Bone Joint Surg Am 1973;55(7): 1331–50.

43. Flandry F, Hommel G. Normal anatomy and biomechanics of the knee. Sports Med Arthrosc Rev 2011; 19(2):82–92.

44. Noyes FR, Grood ES, Torzilli PA. Current concepts review. The definitions of terms for motion and position of the knee and injuries of the ligaments. J Bone Joint Surg Am 1989;71(3):465–72.

45. Moatshe G, Dornan GJ, Ludvigsen T, et al. High prevalence of knee osteoarthritis at a minimum 10-year follow-up after knee dislocation surgery. Knee Surg Sports Traumatol Arthrosc 2017;25(12): 3914–22.

46. Delamarter RB, Hohl M, Hopp E Jr. Ligament injuries associated with tibial plateau fractures. Clin Orthop Relat Res 1990;(250):226–33.

47. Johnson RJ, Kettelkamp DB, Clark W, et al. Factors effecting late results after meniscectomy. J Bone Joint Surg Am 1974;56(4):719–29.

48. Jensen DB, Rude C, Duus B, et al. Tibial plateau fractures. A comparison of conservative and surgical treatment. J Bone Joint Surg Br 1990;72(1): 49–52.

49. Forman JM, Karia RJ, Davidovitch RI, et al. Tibial plateau fractures with and without meniscus tear—results of a standardized treatment protocol. Bull Hosp Jt Dis (2013) 2013;71(2):144–51.

50. Schatzker J, McBroom R, Bruce D. The tibial plateau fracture. The Toronto experience 1968–1975. Clin Orthop Relat Res 1979;(138):94–104.

51. Chang H, Zheng Z, Shao D, et al. Incidence and radiological predictors of concomitant meniscal and cruciate ligament injuries in operative tibial plateau fractures: a prospective diagnostic study. Sci Rep 2018;8(1):13317.

52. Gardner MJ, Yacoubian S, Geller D, et al. The incidence of soft tissue injury in operative tibial plateau fractures: a magnetic resonance imaging analysis of 103 patients. J Orthop Trauma 2005; 19(2):79–84.

53. Warner SJ, Garner MR, Schottel PC, et al. The effect of soft tissue injuries on clinical outcomes after tibial plateau fracture fixation. J Orthop Trauma 2018;32(3):141–7.

54. Haller JM, O'Toole R, Graves M, et al. How much articular displacement can be detected using fluoroscopy for tibial plateau fractures? Injury 2015; 46(11):2243–7.

55. Gosling T, Klingler K, Geerling J, et al. Improved intra-operative reduction control using a three-dimensional mobile image intensifier - a proximal tibia cadaver study. Knee 2009;16(1):58–63.

56. Wright RW, Group M. Osteoarthritis classification scales: interobserver reliability and arthroscopic correlation. J Bone Joint Surg Am 2014;96(14): 1145–51.

57. Healy WL, Brooker AF Jr. Distal femoral fractures. Comparison of open and closed methods of treatment. Clin Orthop Relat Res 1983;174: 166–71.

58. Nasr AM, Mc Leod I, Sabboubeh A, et al. Conservative or surgical management of distal femoral fractures. A retrospective study with a minimum five year follow-up. Acta Orthop Belg 2000;66(5): 477–83.

59. Thomson AB, Driver R, Kregor PJ, et al. Long-term functional outcomes after intra-articular distal femur fractures: ORIF versus retrograde intramedullary nailing. Orthopedics 2008;31(8): 748–50.

60. Hoffmann MF, Jones CB, Sietsema DL, et al. Clinical outcomes of locked plating of distal femoral fractures in a retrospective cohort. J Orthop Surg Res 2013;8:43.

61. Harvin WH, Oladeji LO, Della Rocca GJ, et al. Working length and proximal screw constructs in plate osteosynthesis of distal femur fractures. Injury 2017;48(11):2597–601.

62. Wenger D, Andersson S. Low risk of nonunion with lateral locked plating of distal femoral fractures-A retrospective study of 191 consecutive patients. Injury 2019;50(2):448–52.

63. Lewis SL, Pozo JL, Muirhead-Allwood WF. Coronal fractures of the lateral femoral condyle. J Bone Joint Surg Br 1989;71(1):118–20.

64. Nork SE, Segina DN, Aflatoon K, et al. The association between supracondylar-intercondylar distal femoral fractures and coronal plane fractures. J Bone Joint Surg Am 2005;87(3):564–9.

65. Telleria JJ, Barei DP, Nork SE. Coronal plane small-fragment fixation in supracondylar intercondylar femur fractures. Orthopedics 2016;39(1):e134–9.

66. Starr AJ, Jones AL, Reinert CM. The "swashbuckler": a modified anterior approach for fractures of the distal femur. J Orthop Trauma 1999;13(2):138–40.

67. Espinoza-Ervin CZ, Starr AJ, Reinert CM, et al. Use of a midline anterior incision for isolated medial tibial plateau fractures. J Orthop Trauma 2009;23(2):148–53.

68. Gonzalez LJ, Lott A, Konda S, et al. The Hyperextension Tibial Plateau Fracture Pattern: A Predictor of Poor Outcome. J Orthop Trauma 2017;31(11):e369–74.

69. Caspari RB, Hutton PM, Whipple TL, et al. The role of arthroscopy in the management of tibial plateau fractures. Arthroscopy 1985;1(2):76–82.

70. Jennings JE. Arthroscopic management of tibial plateau fractures. Arthroscopy 1985;1(3):160–8.

71. Burdin G. Arthroscopic management of tibial plateau fractures: surgical technique. Orthop Traumatol Surg Res 2013;99(1 Suppl):S208–18.

72. Chen XZ, Liu CG, Chen Y, et al. Arthroscopy-assisted surgery for tibial plateau fractures. Arthroscopy 2015;31(1):143–53.

73. Liporace FA, Yoon RS. Nail plate combination technique for native and periprosthetic distal femur fractures. J Orthop Trauma 2019;33(2):e64–8.

74. Smith JR, Halliday R, Aquilina AL, et al. Distal femoral fractures: the need to review the standard of care. Injury 2015;46(6):1084–8.

75. Rosen AL, Strauss E. Primary total knee arthroplasty for complex distal femur fractures in elderly patients. Clin Orthop Relat Res 2004;425:101–5.

76. Appleton P, Moran M, Houshian S, et al. Distal femoral fractures treated by hinged total knee replacement in elderly patients. J Bone Joint Surg Br 2006;88(8):1065–70.

77. Bettin CC, Weinlein JC, Toy PC, et al. Distal femoral replacement for acute distal femoral fractures in elderly patients. J Orthop Trauma 2016;30(9):503–9.

78. Weinlein JC, Ford MC, Heck RK. Arthroplasty for older patients with fractures about the knee. In: Borrelli JA Jr, Anglen JO, editors. Arthroplasty for the treatment of fracture in the older patient. Springer International Publishing; 2018. p. 183–98.

79. Haufe T, Forch S, Muller P, et al. The role of a primary arthroplasty in the treatment of proximal tibia fractures in orthogeriatric patients. Biomed Res Int 2016;2016:6047876.

80. Streubel PN, Ricci WM, Wong A, et al. Mortality after distal femur fractures in elderly patients. Clin Orthop Relat Res 2011;469(4):1188–96.

81. Konda SR, Pean CA, Goch AM, et al. Comparison of short-term outcomes of geriatric distal femur and femoral neck fractures: results from the NSQIP database. Geriatr Orthop Surg Rehabil 2015;6(4):311–5.

82. Pearse EO, Klass B, Bendall SP, et al. Stanmore total knee replacement versus internal fixation for supracondylar fractures of the distal femur in elderly patients. Injury 2005;36(1):163–8.

83. Hart GP, Kneisl JS, Springer BD, et al. Open reduction vs distal femoral replacement arthroplasty for comminuted distal femur fractures in the patients 70 years and older. J Arthroplasty 2017;32(1):202–6.

84. Wasserstein D, Henry P, Paterson JM, et al. Risk of total knee arthroplasty after operatively treated tibial plateau fracture: a matched-population-based cohort study. J Bone Joint Surg Am 2014;96(2):144–50.

85. Weiss NG, Parvizi J, Hanssen AD, et al. Total knee arthroplasty in post-traumatic arthrosis of the knee. J Arthroplasty 2003;18(3 Suppl 1):23–6.

86. Larson AN, Hanssen AD, Cass JR. Does prior infection alter the outcome of TKA after tibial plateau fracture? Clin Orthop Relat Res 2009;467(7):1793–9.

87. Saleh H, Yu S, Vigdorchik J, et al. Total knee arthroplasty for treatment of post-traumatic arthritis: systematic review. World J Orthop 2016;7(9):584–91.

88. Papadopoulos EC, Parvizi J, Lai CH, et al. Total knee arthroplasty following prior distal femoral fracture. Knee 2002;9(4):267–74.

89. Martin-Hernandez C, Floria-Arnal LJ, Gomez-Blasco A, et al. Metaphyseal sleeves as the primary implant for the management of bone defects in total knee arthroplasty after post-traumatic knee arthritis. Knee 2018;25(4):669–75.

90. Abdel MP, von Roth P, Cross WW, et al. Total knee arthroplasty in patients with a prior tibial plateau fracture: a long-term report at 15 years. J Arthroplasty 2015;30(12):2170–2.

91. Bajaj S, Shoemaker T, Hakimiyan AA, et al. Protective effect of P188 in the model of acute trauma to human ankle cartilage: the mechanism of action. J Orthop Trauma 2010;24(9):571–6.

92. Chang JC, Christiansen BA, Murugesh DK, et al. SOST/sclerostin improves posttraumatic osteoarthritis and inhibits MMP2/3 expression after injury. J Bone Miner Res 2018;33(6):1105–13.

93. Mishra A, Srivastava RN, Awasthi S, et al. Expression of genes and their polymorphism influences the risk of knee osteoarthritis. J Nucleic Acids 2017;2017:3138254.

94. Pizanis A, Garcia P, Pohlemann T, et al. Balloon tibioplasty: a useful tool for reduction of tibial plateau depression fractures. J Orthop Trauma 2012;26(7):e88–93.

Pediatrics

Pediatric Septic Arthritis
An Update

Daniel W. Brown, MD[a], Benjamin W. Sheffer, MD[b],*

KEYWORDS

- Septic arthritis • Osteoarticular infection • Pyogenic arthritis • Children

KEY POINTS

- Septic arthritis in children is a surgical emergency and prompt diagnosis is mandatory.
- Careful history, physical examination, imaging, and laboratory testing are required for accurate diagnosis.
- Immediate irrigation and débridement of the joint followed by antibiotics are the keys of treatment.
- With prompt diagnosis and appropriate treatment, results generally are very good, with few long-term sequelae.
- Delay in diagnosis and treatment can result in growth disturbance and joint destruction.

Septic arthritis in children occurs with varying rates depending on a child's age and situation. The peak age of infection ranges from younger than 2 years to 6 years, with an incidence of 4 to 10 per 100,000 in well-resourced countries.[1] In low-income countries, an incidence of 5 to 20 per 100,000 children has been reported.[2] Controversy exists as to whether infection rates are increasing or decreasing.[3] Hospitalization rates due to septic arthritis among children are decreasing, with the highest rates of hospitalization in children ages 0 to 4 years who live in low-income areas, even in a well-resourced country.[4] The large joints of the lower extremities are most commonly affected, with up to 80% of cases involving the hip or knee[5]; however, any joint can be infected from the shoulder or elbow to even the facet joints of the spine.[1,5,6] Osteomyelitis and bacteremia/septicemia are significantly associated with an infection of a large joint in children 10 years to 14 years of age.[4]

ETIOLOGY

Primary septic arthritis is a result of hematogenous (most common) or direct inoculation.[7] Secondary septic arthritis occurs when nearby infection spreads to the joint. This most commonly occurs when osteomyelitis in intra-articular metaphyseal bone breaks through the cortex into the joint and seeds it. Joints at risk for this include the shoulder, elbow, hip, and ankle but not the knee. Although much less common, infection also can spread in the opposite direction, with primary infection of the joint leading to penetration of the epiphyseal cartilage and then to the metaphysis through the transphyseal vessels, which are present during the first 12 months to 18 months of life.[8] Once present in the joint, bacterial toxins and a cascade of cytokines from damaged tissue activate what has collectively been referred to as the acute-phase response.[9] These enzymes from damaged tissue and responding leukocytes, as well as bacterial toxins, can lead to articular cartilage damage in as little as 8 hours.[10,11] Ongoing infection and tissue injury can be considered continuous activation of the acute phase response, only halted by initiation of antibiotic therapy or surgical débridement.[9]

Disclosure Statement: The authors have nothing to disclose.
[a] Department of Orthopaedic Surgery and Biomedical Engineering, Le Bonheur Children's Hospital, University of Tennessee–Campbell Clinic, 1211 Union Avenue, Suite 520, Memphis, TN 38104, USA; [b] Campbell Clinic, 7545 Airways Blvd, Southaven, MS 38671, USA
* Corresponding author.
E-mail address: bsheffer@campbellclinic.com

BACTERIOLOGY

The most commonly isolated bacteria in septic arthritis across all age groups continues to be *Staphylococcus aureus*, both methicillin-sensitive *S aureus* and methicillin-resistant *S aureus* (MRSA).[12] Much has been written about the mecA gene that confers this antibiotic resistance to β-lactam antibiotics and the Panton-Valentine leukocidin gene locus that enables certain strains of hospital-acquired and community-acquired *S aureus* to produce cytotoxin and cause tissue necrosis.[13] Rates of infection caused by either MRSA or group A β-hemolytic streptococcus are increasing and lead to a more difficult and dangerous clinical course.[14,15] *Kingella kingae* should be considered, particularly in children younger than 4 years of age[16] and older than 3 months. In infants, group B streptococcus is most common, but several other organisms have been reported in infants and older children (Table 1).[17–22]

DIAGNOSIS

Prompt diagnosis is vital for favorable outcomes and is based on the entirety of patient history, physical examination, imaging, laboratory studies, and aspiration of the suspected joint.

Presentation/History

Medical advice usually is sought within 2 days to 6 days of the onset of symptoms,[23] which generally include an acute onset of pain, swelling, immobility of the joint,[17] and, in the lower extremities, refusal to bear weight.[24] Fever may or may not be reported. Often there is a history of an innocuous injury or fall. Infants may present with only malaise or listlessness.[7] A thorough history must be taken and should include age, prematurity, recent procedures, medications, travel history, sick contacts (or even contacts with young children), immunization status, recent illnesses, animal exposures, and exposure to unpasteurized dairy products.[25] Heightened suspicion is needed because these patients can be a diagnostic dilemma. One study reported the initial emergency department diagnosis to be consistent with the definitive diagnosis only 42% of the time.[26]

Physical Examination

The hip is the most commonly affected joint, followed by the knee.[1] The affected joint is irritable

Table 1 Bacteriology		
Bacteriology of septic arthritis		
S aureus	Most common across all age groups	
K kingae	Children younger than 4 y and older than 3 mo	
Group B streptococcus	Most common in infants[17,18]	
Haemophilus influenza		
Streptococcus pneumoniae		
Salmonella enterica		
Klebsiella pneumonia		
Candida albicans		
Less common causative organisms		
Pseudomonas aeruginosa	Suspected in penetrating foot wounds but has been reported without the initiating trauma[19]	
Pasteurella canis	Most often after animal bites but has been found without animal contact[20]	
Salmonella typhi	Suspected in children with sickle cell disease or trait but has been found in immunocompetent children[21]	
Neisseria gonorrhoeae	Suspected in sexually active adolescents but may be present in cases of sexual abuse[6]	
H influenza	Rare, due to vaccinations for type B, but has been reported in unvaccinated populations and populations at risk for non–type B serotypes[22]	

and is most often held in a position of comfort, one that maximizes intracapsular volume. In the hip this position is flexed, abducted, and externally rotated.[27] Other clinical features may include effusion, erythema, heat, tenderness to palpation, and, in the lower extremities, inability to bear weight or altered gait. The more superficial the joint, the more readily apparent these features are. Perhaps the most useful sign is micromotion tenderness.[28] A retrospective review of children with MRSA septic arthritis demonstrated that 63% had a temperature over 38.5°C at presentation.[29] When vital sign disturbances are seen, the child is ill or toxic appearing, or multiple sites are involved, a more virulent organism, advanced course, or disseminated infection is present.[1]

Imaging

Historically, radiographs of the involved joint were recommended as the first line of imaging in suspected articular infection.[7,25] They remain an inexpensive and rapid imaging modality. In the acute setting, they often are normal because infection may require 7 days to 10 days before bony changes become apparent.[7] Additionally, in very young patients, the ossific nucleus may not have formed, further limiting radiographic yield. Because of this limited utility and exposure to radiation, recent investigations have questioned their routine use.[30] Because other conditions, however, such as trauma or tumor, can present with joint pain, radiographs are still helpful to rule out some of those conditions. Radiographic findings include soft tissue swelling and joint space widening in the short term. Long-term changes include periosteal reaction, osteolysis, and joint space narrowing.[7,25]

Ultrasound is a safe (no radiation or sedation and noninvasive) and easily conducted examination to confirm an effusion.[31] It also is rapid and inexpensive. It cannot, however, distinguish between sterile, purulent, and hemorrhagic fluid accumulations.[32] An effusion on ultrasound paired with high clinical suspicion of septic arthritis warrants aspiration, for which ultrasound may be used as an aid (**Fig. 1**). Some investigators recommend proceeding directly to arthrotomy and débridement.[31] A negative ultrasound of the hip with an absence of fluid generally rules

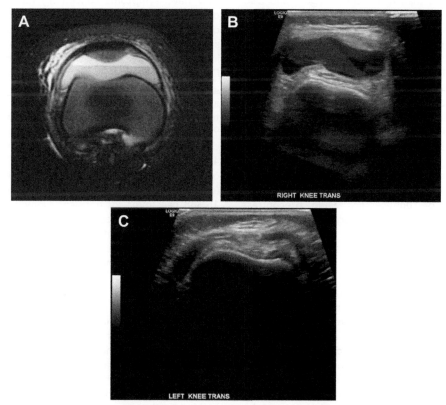

Fig. 1. (A) Axial T2 MRI of a 16-month-old boy with culture-positive septic arthritis of the right knee. (B) Corresponding ultrasound image shows large effusion and fluid level. (C) For comparison, the ultrasound of the unaffected contralateral knee shows no effusion.

out septic arthritis.[25] A downside to ultrasound is that it can be very user-dependent, and it does not necessarily rule out nearby osteomyelitis or intramuscular abscess. Because concurrent osteomyelitis and septic arthritis are frequent, some investigators have recommended magnetic resonance imaging (MRI) in cases of suspected musculoskeletal infection,[33] whereas others acknowledge that MRI can be ordered unnecessarily[34] and recommend following the clinical course for response to treatment before ordering an MRI.[31]

If a diagnosis remains unclear, MRI can demonstrate the full extent of the infection to correctly guide treatment.[35] A prime example of this is using MRI to distinguish septic arthritis of the hip from a psoas abscess. Because MRI is costly and may not be readily available in some centers, algorithms to guide appropriate use have been developed (**Fig. 2**)[36] but may[37] or may not[38] be applicable to all patient populations. Certain body regions, such as the elbow[12] and shoulder,[38,39] have high incidences of concurrent osteomyelitis, and MRI evaluation should be considered in the evaluation of these joints. MRI also has shown increased utility in young children less than 4 months of age[39] and also can show perfusion in the hip, which can highlight risk for future secondary osteomyelitis or ischemic necrosis.[8] The drawbacks of MRI are the cost, time required to obtain, and need for sedation in certain patients. In an effort at efficiency and diagnostic accuracy, some centers have made agreements with their radiology department to obtain a single-sequence MRI within a timely manner (within 1 hour), usually a coronal plane T2 or short-tau inversion recovery image of the affected region. Bilateral imaging has not been shown to alter treatment.[40] Gadolinium contrast-enhanced MRI has been indicated to be unnecessary when precontrast images are normal,[41] although some investigators contend that this is the reason contrast is needed.[42]

Laboratory Studies

In addition to vital signs, standard laboratory studies should be ordered, including complete blood cell count with differential, basic serum chemistry, C-reactive protein (CRP), erythrocyte sedimentation rate (ESR), and blood cultures.[13] It is vital that blood cultures be obtained before initiation of antibiotics. The Kocher criteria (white blood cell [WBC] count >12,000 cells/μL of serum, inability to bear weight, fever >101.3° F [38.5°C], and ESR >40 mm/ h),[42] originally described for the hip to distinguish infection from synovitis, has been applied to other joints.[43] In practice, however, CRP, a nonspecific marker of inflammation, has been shown more useful than ESR because of its shorter half-life, especially to follow response to treatment.[44] Determining a cutoff for CRP is difficult.[45,46] A more virulent organism (MRSA) or concurrent adjacent osteomyelitis each can lead to a much higher elevation in CRP than transient synovitis or infection by K kingae, for example. In addition, reference ranges for CRP vary by institution and publication.

Serum procalcitonin is a promising acute-phase reactant that may be more useful than CRP,[47] but further research is needed before its routine clinical use.[9]

Differential Diagnosis

The differential is large, and treatment often is begun empirically. During the evaluation of the patient, various diagnoses should be ruled out. In addition to history and physical examination, plain radiographs and ultrasound should eliminate fracture and other structural diagnoses, such as (in the hip) slipped capital femoral epiphysis or Legg-Calvé-Perthes disease. In patients who have symptoms concerning for leukemia or sickle cell crisis, a peripheral blood smear differentiates. An MRI, if obtained, rules out subperiosteal abscess, cellulitis, osteomyelitis, intramuscular abscess or pyomyositis, and tumor. Differentiating among septic arthritis, Lyme arthritis, transient (toxic) synovitis, and juvenile idiopathic arthritis is more difficult. A recent systematic review and meta-analysis showed the 95% CI for ESR was 21 mm/h to 33 mm/h in those diagnosed with transient synovitis, 37 mm/h to 46 mm/h for Lyme arthritis, and 44 mm/h to 64 mm/h for septic arthritis. Synovial WBC count (cells/mm^3) 95% CIs were 5644 cells/mm^3 to 15,388 cells/mm^3 for transient synovitis, 47,533 cells/mm^3 to 64,242 cells/mm^3 for Lyme arthritis, and 105,432 cells/mm^3 to 260,214 cells/mm^3 for septic arthritis.[48] In distinguishing juvenile idiopathic arthritis, a nonresponse to treatment may the only distinguishing characteristic.[49] Transient synovitis often is preceded by an upper respiratory infection. The child also has a less severe presentation and likely is afebrile. Juvenile idiopathic arthritis may be polyarticular and migratory and likely has a subacute onset at presentation. The child also may have a rash.[7] The difficulty in distinguishing between Lyme arthritis and septic arthritis from a low virulence organism highlights the need to obtain serologies in endemic areas and culture or PCR for K kingae in appropriate age groups.

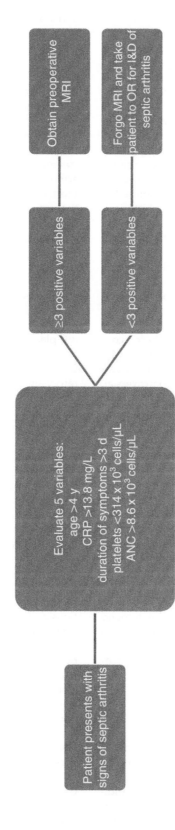

Fig. 2. Flowchart for the proposed algorithm for determining whether patients with septic arthritis should have preoperative MRI. ANC, absolute neutrophil count. I&D, Incision and Drainage; OR, Operating Room. (*From* Rosenfeld S, Bernstein DT, Daram S, et al. Predicting the presence of adjacent infections in septic arthritis in children. J Pediatr Orthop 2016;36(1):74; with permission.)

Aspirate

Aspiration is essential for suspected but unproved infections and should be done before antibiotic administration; it can be done in the operating room at the time of surgery. Cloudy, turbid, and purulent fluid that has lost the string sign favors the diagnosis. Synovial fluid analysis should be performed, including cell count with differential, Gram stain, glucose, and anaerobic and aerobic cultures.[25] Antibiotic susceptibility also should be ordered. In children 4 years of age and younger, because of their high risk for *K kingae*, synovial fluid should be injected directly into blood culture vials to reduce the rate of culture negative results for this historically difficult to culture organism[50,51] or sent for polymerase chain reaction (PCR), if available. Recent studies have questioned the relevance of routine Gram stain use.[52] Additional work has recommended that the ilium and proximal femur also be aspirated at the time of hip aspiration in the OR to increase culture sensitivity.[53] Femoral neck aspiration at the time of surgery has been shown to increase sensitivity for concurrent osteomyelitis, particularly when the MRI is falsely negative.[54] Synovial fluid analysis and cut-off for infection continue to be controversial, with 1 recent review recommending a WBC count of greater than 50,000/mm³ and greater than 75% polymorphonuclear (PMN) cells[25] (and another recommending WBC count greater than 100,000/mm³ and >90% PMN cells).[7]

If available, PCR of synovial fluid or tissue can speed up identification of the organism, assist with difficult to culture organisms, such as *K kingae*, and in cases where antibiotics have been started.[7] Depending on laboratory set up, time to results, although previously reported at 5 days,[55] has been reduced to less than 24 hours.[56] Different variations exist, including multiplex, 16S, real-time, and gram typing. As research has progressed, different loci that were thought to be diagnostic have been found to exist in multiple strains.[57] PCR remains a promising area of research that likely will have an increasing impact in the future. In endemic regions, a Lyme titer and PCR also should be sent as Lyme Disease remains on the differential.[7]

TREATMENT

Treatment of septic arthritis is best carried out in a well-coordinated multidisciplinary manner.[13] Prompt diagnosis, treatment, pain control, and rehabilitation can lead to good results. In addition to those discussed previously, recent studies showed the addition of a short course of dexamethasone to lead to earlier clinical and laboratory improvement.[58,59] This is a promising avenue, with more work to be done in the future.[60]

Operative Treatment

Timely drainage, decompression, irrigation, and débridement remain the hallmarks of surgical treatment. Decompression is particularly important in the hip because it is at risk for osteonecrosis. Open arthrotomy has been the mainstay of treatment, but recent studies have shown arthroscopy to be a successful alternative in the knee,[61] hip,[62] ankle, and shoulder, even in the very young.[63] Patients who had arthroscopic débridement of the knee ranged the knee 5 days and walked 7 days sooner than those who had open surgery, but there were no long-term differences.[64] Risk of revision surgery is associated with older children, a delay in diagnosis, markedly elevated CRP at presentation and continued on postoperative days 1 through 4, and positive blood cultures.[65] Drains frequently are placed in both arthroscopic and open procedures and usually removed 2 or 3 days after surgery. If drainage persists, no clinical or laboratory improvement is made, repeat irrigation and débridement should be undertaken, and repeat MRI considered. Serial operations are warranted until there is clinical improvement.

Antibiotics

Antibiotic treatment typically begins with broad coverage that is narrowed as soon as aspirate or surgical cultures allow. Antibiotics should be started after blood cultures and synovial fluid samples have been obtained. Most Surgeons argue that antibiotics should be delayed until operative irrigation and débridement have been performed so adequate samples can be obtained for culture.[66] Ideally, the choice of antibiotic should be made in conjunction with the infectious disease service.[25] Once clinical and laboratory progress is made, the patient is transitioned to oral antibiotics. The length of treatment has been to be reported as short as 10 days of oral antibiotics in simple cases,[67] although the ideal length of treatment has not been determined.[1]

Initial starting antibiotics typically are a first-generation cephalosporin or penicillinase-resistance penicillin from Gram-positive coverage, such as staphylococcus or streptococcal species. Vancomycin or clindamycin are added in areas with high MRSA prevalence. Care must be taken with clindamycin because resistance can be induced in MRSA[23] by enzymatic methylation of the antibiotic binding site in the 50S ribosomal subunit.[68] If *K kingae*, Lyme disease, or *Neisseria gonorrhoeae* is suspected, a third-generation cephalosporin, such as ceftriaxone, is more effective.[25] Duration of intravenous therapy in simple cases often is 4 days, and, once susceptibilities return, the patient is placed on oral antibiotics for 2 weeks to 4 weeks.[23]

Serial Aspiration

Because of the morbidity of open arthrotomy, particularly in simple isolated cases, or in patients for whom surgery is contraindicated, therapeutic aspiration remains an option. In 1 study with good outcomes at an average follow-up of 7.4 years, 42 children with septic arthritis of the hip who were successfully treated by serial aspiration and lavage with normal saline (N = 33) had a mean age of 2.6 years, whereas those who required surgery (N = 9) had a mean age of 8.3 years. In this study, the indication for aspiration was a joint effusion of 5 mm or more on ultrasound, and ultrasound examination was repeated daily until discharge.[69] In another study, all 17 children with septic arthritis of the hip were treated successfully with serial aspirations and were doing well with up to 4 years of follow-up.[70] A recent study identified risk factors for failure of aspiration as a treatment of septic arthritis of the knee as age greater than 3 years and CRP of more than 20 mg/L.[71] Although it may require more than one aspiration, it is a viable option in young patients.

OUTCOMES

If the diagnosis is made promptly and treatment is begun in a timely manner, the outcome can be very good. Patients can make dramatic improvement, return to previous levels of function quickly, and have few long-term sequelae; however, with a delay in diagnosis and treatment, or the presence of a virulent organism, the outcomes can range from growth disturbance and joint destruction[72] (**Fig. 3**) to septic emboli, deep vein thrombosis, multiorgan system failure, and even death. Historically, rates of complications approached 50% but more recently have been as low as 10%.[73] Long-term monitoring is indicated,[74] especially of patients with infection near growth centers.[13] In uncomplicated cases, patients may be kept weight bearing as tolerated and the hospital stay limited to 3 to 4 days. This allows time for cultures to result, transition from intravenous to oral antibiotics to occur and clinical and laboratory improvement to be observed.

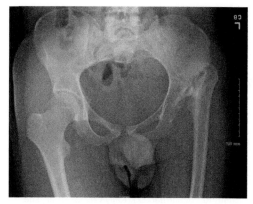

Fig. 3. Anteroposterior radiograph of a 17-year-old boy with chronic left hip pain as a sequel of missed septic arthritis as an infant.

SUMMARY

Septic arthritis in pediatric patients is a challenging entity with a broad differential diagnosis, but it remains a surgical emergency. Many emerging technologies aid in the diagnosis, but evolving bacteria resistance continues to make this a difficult problem to treat. Even so, the diagnosis must be made quickly and treatment begun promptly with surgical irrigation and debridement followed by administration of antibiotics to minimize sequelae in this vulnerable population.

REFERENCES

1. Arnold JC, Bradley JS. Osteoarticular infections in children. Infect Dis Clin North Am 2015;29:557–74.
2. Chiappini E, Mastrolia MV, Galli L, et al. Septic arthritis in children in resource limited and non-resource limited countries: an update on diagnosis and treatment. Expert Rev Anti Infect Ther 2016;14:1087–96.
3. Dodwell ER. Osteomyelitis and septic arthritis in children: current concepts. Curr Opin Pediatr 2013;25:58–63.
4. Okubo Y, Nochioka K, Marcia T. Nationwide survey of pediatric septic arthritis in the United States. J Orthop 2017;14(3):342–6.
5. French R, Purushothaman B, Roysam GS, et al. Pediatric facet joint septic arthritis. Spine J 2015;16:1686–8.
6. Arkader A, Brusalis CM, Warner WC Jr, et al. Update in pediatric musculoskeletal infections: when it is, when it isnt't, and what to do. Instr Course Lect 2017;66:495–504.
7. Le Hanneur M, Vidal C, Mallet C, et al. Unusual case of paediatric septic arthritis of the lumbar facet joints due to Kingella kingae. Orthop Traumatol Surg Res 2016;102:959–61.

8. Merlini L, Anooshiravani M, Ceroni D. Concomitant septic arthritis and osteomyelitis of the hip in young children; a new pathophysiological hypothesis suggested by MRI enhance pattern. BMC Med Imaging 2015;15:17.

9. Benvenuti M, An T, Amaro E, et al. Double-edged sword: musculoskeletal infection provoked acute phase response in children. Orthop Clin North Am 2017;48:181–97.

10. Papathanasiou I, Malizos KN, Poultsides L, et al. The catabolic role of toll-like receptor 2 (TLR-2) mediated by the NF-kB pathway in septic arthritis. J Orthop Res 2011;29:247–51.

11. Smith RL, Schurman DJ, Kajiyama G, et al. The effect of antibiotics on the destruction of cartilage in experimental infectious arthritis. J Bone Joint Surg Am 1987;69:1063–8.

12. Nduaguba AM, Flynn JM, Sankar WN. Septic arthritis of the elbow in children: clinical presentation and microbiological profile. J Pediatr Orthop 2016;36:75–9.

13. Pendletonn A, Kocher MS. Methicillin-resistant staphylococcus aureus bone and joint infections in children. J Am Acad Orthop Surg 2015;23:29–37.

14. Branson J, Vallejo JG, Flores AR, et al. The contemporary microbiology and rates of concomitant osteomyelitis in acute septic arthritis. Pediatr Infect Dis J 2017;36:267–73.

15. Sarkissian EJ, Gans I, Gunderson MA, et al. Community-acquired methicillin-resistant staphylococcu aureus musculoskeletal infections: emerging trends over the past decade. J Pediatr Orthop 2016;36:323–7.

16. Williams N, Cooper C, Cundy P. Kingella kingae septic arthritis in children: recognizing an elusive pathogen. J Child Orthop 2014;8:91–5.

17. Bono KT, Samora JB, Klingele KE. Septic arthritis in infants younger than 3 months: a retrospective review. Orthopedics 2015;38(9):e787–93.

18. Sankaran G, Zacharia B, Roy A, et al. Current clinical and bacteriological profile of septic arthritis in young infants: a prospective study from a tertiary referral centre. Eur J Orthop Surg Traumatol 2018;28(4):573–8.

19. Hatakenaka T, Uemura K, Itsubo T, et al. Septic arthritis of the elbow in a child due to Pseudomonas aeruginosa: a case report. J Pediatr Orthop B 2014;23(3):285–7.

20. Hazelton BJ, Axt MW, Jones CA. Pasteurella canis osteoarticular infections in childhood: review of bone and joint infections due to pasteurella species over 10 years at a tertiary pediatric hospital and in the literature. J Pediatr Orthop 2013;33(3):e34–8.

21. Balakumara B, Gangadharan S, Ponmudi N, et al. Atypical osteomyelitis and concurrent septic arthritis due to Salmonella in immunocompetent children. J Clin Orthop Trauma 2017;8(3):293–7.

22. Pavlik DF, Johnston JJ, Eldredge JD, et al. Non-type b haemophilus influenzae septic arthritis in children. J Pediatric Infect Dis Soc 2017;6(3):e134–9.

23. Pääkkönen M, Peltola H. Treatment of acute septic arthritis. Pediatr Infect Dis J 2013;32:684–5.

24. Dartnell J, Ramachandran M, Katchburian M. Haematogenous acute and subacute paediatric osteomyelitis: a systematic review of the literature. J Bone Joint Surg Br 2012;94:584–95.

25. Montgomery NI, Epps HR. Pediatric septic arthritis. Orthop Clin North Am 2017;48:209–16.

26. Vardiabasis NV, Schlechter JA. Definitive diagnosis of children presenting to a pediatric emergency department with fever and extremity pain. J Emerg Med 2017;53:306–12.

27. Naranje S, Kelly DM, Sawyer JR. A systematic approach to the evaluation of a limping child. Am Fam Physician 2015;92:908–16.

28. Baldwin KD, Brusalis CM, Nduaguba AM, et al. Predictive factors for differentiating between septic arthritis and Lyme disease of the knee in children. J Bone Joint Surg Am 2016;98:721–8.

29. Vander Have KL, Karmazyn B, Verma M, et al. Community-associated methicillin-resistant Staphylococcu aureus in acute musculoskeletal infection in children: a game changer. J Pediatr Orthop 2009;29:927–31.

30. Manz N, Krieg AH, Heininger U, et al. Evaluation of the current use of imaging modalities and pathogen detection in children with acute osteomyelitis and septic arthritis. Eur J Pediatr 2018;177:1071–80.

31. Laine JC, Denning JR, Riccio AI, et al. The use of ultrasound in the management of septic arthritis of the hip. J Pediatr Orthop B 2015;24:95–8.

32. Milla SS, Coley BD, Karmazyn B, et al. ACR appropriateness criteria® limping child—ages 0-5 years. J Am Coll Radiol 2012;9:545–53.

33. Monsalve J, Kan JH, Schallert EK, et al. Septic arthritis in children: frequency of coexisting unsuspected osteomyelitis and implications on imaging work-up and management. AJR Am J Roentgenol 2015;204:1289–95.

34. Refakis CA, Arkader A, Baldwin KD, et al. Predicting periarticular infection in children with septic arthritis of the hip: regionally derived criteria may not apply to all populations. J Pediatr Orthop 2019;39(5):268–74.

35. Song KS, Lee SW, Bae KC. Key role of magnetic resonance imaging in the diagnosis of infections around the hip and pelvic girdle mimicking septic arthritis of the hip in children. J Pediatr Orthop B 2016;25:234–40.

36. Rosenfeld S, Bernstein DT, Daram S, et al. Predicting the presence of adjacent infections in septic arthritis in children. J Pediatr Orthop 2016;36:70–4.

37. Welling BD, Haruno LS, Rosenfeld SB. Validating an algorithm to predict adjacent musculoskeletal infections in pediatric patients with septic arthritis. Clin Orthop Relat Res 2018;476:153–9.

38. Emat J, Riccio AI, Fitzpatrick K, et al. Osteomyelitis is commonly associated with septic arthritis of the shoulder in children. J Pediatr Orthop 2017;37:547–52.

39. Montgomery CO, Siegel E, Blasier RD, et al. Concurrent septic arthritis and osteomyelitis in children. J Pediatr Orthop 2013;33:464–7.

40. Metwalli ZA, Kan JH, Munjal KA, et al. MRI of suspected lower extremity musculoskeletal infection in the pediatric patient: how useful is bilateral imaging? AJR Am J Roentgenol 2013;201:427–32.

41. Kan JH, Young RS, Yu C, et al. Clinical impact of gadolinium in the MRI diagnosis of musculoskeletal infection in children. Pediatr Radiol 2010;40:1197–205.

42. Browne LP, Guillerman RP, Orth RC, et al. Community-acquired staphylococcal musculoskeletal infection in infants and young children: necessity of contrast-enhanced MRI for the diagnosis of growth cartilage involvement. AJR Am J Roentgenol 2012;198:194–9.

43. Obey MR, Minaie A, Schipper JA, et al. Pediatric septic arthritis: predictors of septic hip do not apply. J Pediatr Orthop 2019. [Epub ahead of print].

44. Chou AC, Mahadev A. The use of C-reactive protein as a guide for transitioning to oral antibiotics in pediatric osteoarticular infections. J Pediatr Orthop 2016;36:173–7.

45. Rutz E, Spoerri M. Septic arthritis of the paediatric hip – a review of current diagnostic approaches and therapeutic concepts. Acta Orthop Belg 2013;79:123–34.

46. Bernstein DT, Haruno LS, Daram S, et al. Patient factors associated with methicillin-resistant staphylococcus aureus septic arthritis in children. Orthopedics 2018;41:e277–82.

47. Zhao J, Zhang S, Zhang L, et al. Serum procalcitonin levels as a diagnostic marker for septic arthritis: a meta-analysis. Am J Emerg Med 2017;35:1166–71.

48. Cruz AI Jr, Anari JB, Ramirez JM, et al. Distinguishing pediatric Lyme arthritis of the hip from transient synovitis and acute bacterial septic arthritis: a systematic review and meta-analysis. Cureus 2018;10:e2112.

49. Aupiais C, Basmaci R, Ilharreborde B, et al. Arthritis in children: comparison of clinical and biological characteristics of septic arthritis and juvenile idiopathic arthritis. Arch Dis Child 2017;102:316–22.

50. Yagupsky P. Microbiological diagnosis of skeletal system infections in children. Curr Pediatr Rev 2019. [Epub ahead of print].

51. Yagupsky P. Kingella kingae: carriage, transmission, and disease. Clin Microbiol Rev 2015;28:54–79.

52. Bram JT, Baldwin KD, Blumberg JT. Gram stain is not clinically relevant in treatment of pediatric septic arthritis. J Pediatr Orthop 2018;38:e536–40.

53. Schmale GA, Bompadre V. Aspirations of the ilium and proximal femur increase the likelihood of culturing an organism in patients with presumed septic arthritis of the hip. J Child Orthop 2015;9:313–8.

54. Schlung JE, Bastrom TP, Roocroft JH, et al. Femoral neck aspiration aids in the diagnosis of osteomyelitis in children with septic hip. J Pediatr Orthop 2018;38:532–6.

55. Carter K, Doern C, Jo CH, et al. The clinical usefulness of polymerase chain reaction as a supplemental diagnostic tool in the evaluation and the treatment of children with septic arthritis. J Pediatr Orthop 2016;36:167–72.

56. Yagupsky P. Diagnosing Kingella kingae infections in infants and young children. Expert Rev Anti Infect Ther 2017;15:925–34.

57. El Houmami N, Bzdrenga J, Durand GA, et al. Molecular tests that target the RTX locus do not distinguish between Kingella kingae and the recently described Kingella negevensis species. J Clin Microbiol 2017;55:3113–22.

58. Fogel I, Amir J, Bar-On E, et al. Dexamethasone therapy for septic arthritis in children. Pediatrics 2015;136:776–82.

59. Qin YF, Li ZJ, Li H. Corticosteroids as adjunctive therapy with antibiotics in the treatment of children with septic arthritis: a meta-analysis. Drug Des Devel Ther 2018;12:2277–84.

60. Farrow L. A systematic review and meta-analysis regarding the use of corticosteroids in septic arthritis. BMC Musculoskelet Disord 2015;16:241.

61. Agout C, Lakhal W, Fournier J, et al. Arthroscopic treatment of septic arthritis of the knee in children. Orthop Traumatol Surg Res 2015;101(8 Suppl):S333–6.

62. Sanpera I, Raluy-Collado D, Sanpera-Iglesias J. Arthroscopy for hip septic arthritis in children. Orthop Traumatol Surg Res 2016;201:87–9.

63. Thompson RM, Gourineni P. Arthroscopic treatment of septic arthritis in very young children. J Pediatr Orthop 2017;37:e53–7.

64. Johns B, Loewenthal M, Ho E, et al. Arthroscopic versus open treatment for acute septic arthritis of the knee in children. Pediatr Infect Dis J 2018;37:413–8.

65. Telleria JJ, Cotter RA, Bompadre V, et al. Laboratory predictors for risk of revision surgery in pediatric septic arthritis. J Child Orthop 2016;10:247–54.

66. MacLean SB, Timmis C, Evans S, et al. Preoperative antibiotics for septic arthritis in children: delay in

diagnosis. J Orthop Surg (Hong Kong) 2015;23: 80–3.

67. Lorrot M, Gillet Y, Gras Le Guen C, et al. Antibiotic therapy of bone and joint infections in children: proposals of the French Pediatric Infectious Disease Group. Arch Pediatr 2017;24(12S): S36–41.

68. Hodille E, Badiou C, Bouveyron C, et al. Clindamycin suppresses virulence expression in inducible clindamycin-resistant Staphylococcus aureus strains. Ann Clin Microbiol Antimicrob 2018;17:38.

69. Weigl DM, Becker T, Mercado E, et al. Percutaneous aspiration and irrigation technique for the treatment of pediatric septic hip: effectiveness and predictive parameters. J Pediatr Orthop B 2016;25:514–9.

70. Kotlarsky P, Savit I, Kassis I, et al. Treatment of septic hip in a pediatric ED: a retrospective case series analysis. Am J Emerg Med 2016;34:602–5.

71. Benvenuti MA, An TJ, Mignemi ME, et al. Effects of antibiotic timing on culture results and clinical outcomes in pediatric musculoskeletal infection. J Pediatr Orthop 2019;39(3):158–62.

72. Kanojia RK, Gupta S, Kumar A, et al. Closed reduction, osteotomy, and fibular graft are effective in treating pediatric femoral neck pseudarthrosis after infection. Clin Orthop Relat Res 2018;476:1479–90.

73. Howardd-Jones AR, Isaacs D, Gibbons PJ. Twelve-month outcome following septic arthritis in children. J Pediatr Orthop B 2013;22:486–90.

74. Pääkkönen M. Septic arthritis in children: diagnosis and treatment. Pediatric Health Med Ther 2017;8: 65–8.

Juvenile Idiopathic Arthritis for the Pediatric Orthopedic Surgeon

Karen M. Bovid, MD[a],*, Mary D. Moore, MD[b]

KEYWORDS

- Juvenile idiopathic arthritis • Juvenile rheumatoid arthritis • Juvenile chronic arthritis • Enthesitis
- Spondyloarthropathy

KEY POINTS

- Juvenile idiopathic arthritis (JIA) refers to a group of conditions characterized by joint inflammation of unknown etiology lasting longer than 6 weeks in a patient younger than 16 years.
- Medical management to control inflammation and pain under the direction of a pediatric rheumatologist is the mainstay of treatment.
- Pediatric orthopedic surgeons may be the first providers to identify patients with JIA.
- Surgical treatment may be indicated to address deformity, limb length inequality, or end-stage arthritis.
- Careful preoperative planning and perioperative management in consultation with a patient's rheumatologist are important for successful surgical outcomes.

INTRODUCTION

Juvenile idiopathic arthritis (JIA) refers to a group of conditions characterized by joint inflammation of unknown etiology lasting longer than 6 weeks in a patient younger than 16 years of age.[1] Previously, the term juvenile rheumatoid arthritis (JRA) was used, but, because relatively few patients are rheumatoid factor (RF) positive, this term has been replaced to reflect improved understanding of these disorders.[1,2]

Juvenile arthritis is appropriately managed primarily by pediatric rheumatologists with expertise in diagnosis, classification, laboratory evaluation, and the many anti-inflammatory and disease-modifying antirheumatic drug (DMARD) therapies available. These medications have the potential to prevent much of the destructive arthritis that required orthopedic treatment in the past. Even so, there remain patients who may benefit from orthopedic treatment of deformity, limb length inequality, or end-stage arthritis. Also, many patients with JIA, in particular oligoarticular arthritis (62%), are referred initially to orthopedic surgeons prior to referral to pediatric rheumatologists.[3] It is, therefore, important for pediatric orthopedic surgeons to be comfortable with not only the orthopedic treatment and appropriate perioperative management of patients with JIA but also evaluation of children with possible inflammatory arthritis in order to refer them for pediatric rheumatology care.[4]

The International League of Associations for Rheumatology (ILAR) has classified JIA into

Disclosure Statement: The authors have no relationship with a commercial company that has a direct financial interest in subject matter or materials discussed in article or with a company making a competing product, and no other conflicts of interest to disclose.
[a] Department of Orthopaedic Surgery, Western Michigan University Homer Stryker M.D. School of Medicine, 1000 Oakland Drive, Kalamazoo, MI 49008, USA; [b] Department of Pediatrics, Central Michigan University College of Medicine, 1000 Houghton Avenue, Saginaw, MI 48602, USA
* Corresponding author.
E-mail address: karen.bovid@med.wmich.edu

categories of systemic arthritis, oligoarthritis, poly-arthritis (RF negative), polyarthritis (RF positive), psoriatic arthritis, enthesitis-related arthritis, and undifferentiated arthritis (Table 1).[1] The categories are intended to be mutually exclusive in order to allow for research comparisons. The presence of criteria for 1 category, therefore, is noted as an exclusion for each the other categories.[1,4] For example, the presence of psoriasis is an exclusion for all categories except psoriatic arthritis.

SYSTEMIC JUVENILE IDIOPATHIC ARTHRITIS

Systemic-onset JIA is a multisystem disease characterized by fevers and arthritis of 1 or more joints.[1] Additional features include lymphade-nopathy, hepatomegaly, splenomegaly, serositis, and an erythematous rash with salmon-colored macules that often appears with fever and dissipates hours later.[1,5] The serositis most commonly presents as pericarditis with pericardial effusion, but pleuritis or peritonitis also occur.[5] Pericarditis affects 7.6% of patients and may be asymptomatic or result in symptomatic effusion and rarely cardiac tamponade.[6] In the past, this entity was known as Still disease after George Frederic Still's[7] 1897 description of 22 children with arthritis of multiple joints, fevers, lymphadenopathy, splenomegaly, pericarditis, and growth restriction. Still noted that although there were some similarities in the condition to rheumatoid

Table 1
International League of Associations for Rheumatology classification of juvenile idiopathic arthritis

Juvenile Idiopathic Arthritis Category	Description
Systemic arthritis	Arthritis of 1 or more joints with or preceded by fever of 2 wk that is daily for at least 3 d and 1 or more of the following: • Evanescent (nonfixed) erythematous rash • Generalized lymphadenopathy • Hepatomegaly or splenomegaly • Serositis
Oligoarthritis	Arthritis affecting 1–4 joints in first 6 mo of disease • Persistent: affects no more than 4 joints throughout course • Extended: affects >4 joints total after first 6 mo
Polyarthritis (RF negative)	In the first 6 mo of disease • Arthritis affecting ≥5 joints and • RF test negative
Polyarthritis (RF positive)	In the first 6 mo of disease • Arthritis affecting ≥5 joints and • Two positive RF tests ≥3 mo apart
Psoriatic arthritis	Arthritis and psoriasis, or arthritis and 2 or more of the following: • Dactylitis • Nail pitting or onycholysis • Psoriasis in a first-degree relative
Enthesitis-related arthritis	Arthritis and enthesitis, or arthritis or enthesitis and 2 or more of the following: • SI tenderness or inflammatory lumbosacral pain • HLA-B27 positive • Onset of arthritis > 6-year-old boy • Symptomatic anterior uveitis • History of ankylosing spondylitis, enthesitis-related arthritis, sacroiliitis with inflammatory bowel disease, Reiter syndrome, or anterior uveitis in a first-degree relative
Undifferentiated arthritis	Fulfils criteria in no category or 2 or more categories

arthritis in adults, there also were differences that demonstrated this was a distinct entity.[7] The fever typically is at least 39°C and occurs at least once daily (quotidian), often the late afternoon/evening.[5] The most commonly involved joints include the knee (68%), wrist (68%), and ankle (57%).[8] Symptoms of joint pain and stiffness often are worsened after periods of rest and improved with activity. Patients with persistent systemic symptoms 6 months after onset are at increased risk of joint destruction.[9] Arthritis may present several weeks after fever, which may make the diagnosis of these systemically ill patients difficult. In 1 study, only 30% of patients with systemic JIA met the ILAR criteria at presentation.[8]

A potentially life-threatening complication of systemic JIA is macrophage activation syndrome (MAS), which may be fatal in 20% of cases.[5] MAS has been reported in 7% to 24% of patients with systemic JIA and can occur at any point in the clinical course, even in children with systemic JIA in remission.[10,11] In MAS, overactivation of macrophages and T-lymphocytes leads to an overwhelming inflammatory response. Patients develop mental status changes, cytopenia, mucosal bleeding, and purpura in addition to persistent fever, hepatosplenomegaly with liver dysfunction, and lymphadenopathy. Renal and respiratory failure, hypotension, and shock can occur in severe cases. Laboratory evaluation includes anemia, thrombocytopenia, elevated liver enzymes, lactate dehydrogenase, triglycerides, D-dimer, and ferritin.[5] Disseminated intravascular coagulation may occur. There is a paradoxic decrease in erythrocyte sedimentation rate due to consumption of fibrinogen.[5] Early recognition and treatment of MAS, typically with high-dose methylprednisolone, can be life-saving (Box 1).[5]

OLIGOARTHRITIS

Oligoarticular or pauciarticular JIA is the most common type of JIA[2,4,12] and presents as swelling of 1 to 4 joints. In contrast to systemic-onset JIA, affected children appear well with 1 or a few swollen joints, most commonly involving the knee,[13] ankle, subtalar joint, and elbow in order of decreasing frequency.[2] Only 1 joint is involved in approximately half of patients.[2] The hips, small joints of the hands and feet, and cervical spine usually are not affected.[14] Age of onset typically is before 6 years (peak between ages 2–4)[2] and girls are affected more often than boys by a ratio of 4:1.[4] Joint swelling is caused by a combination of effusion and synovitis and typically is accompanied by comparatively mild pain and tenderness. Patients usually bear weight.[15] Stiffness classically

Box 1
Systemic juvenile idiopathic arthritis case example

A 9-month-old girl was diagnosed with systemic JIA when she presented with fever; rash, polyarthritis involving the hips, knees, shoulders, elbows, wrists, and hands; hepatosplenomegaly; pericarditis; and MAS. She had anemia of chronic disease with hemoglobin ranging from 6.4 g/dL to 9.9 g/dL over the next several years. This was not responsive to treatment with erythropoietin or iron, and she was treated with multiple intermittent blood transfusions for symptomatic anemia. She was admitted to the hospital numerous times with fever and/or anemia. The arthritis and inflammation were difficult to control despite treatment with NSAIDs (ibuprofen, naproxen, and celecoxib), corticosteroids, methotrexate, cyclosporine, cyclophosphamide, TNF inhibitors (infliximab and etanercept), T-lymphocyte inhibitor (abatacept), and IL-1 inhibitor (anakinra). She did have temporary improvement in symptoms of joint pain and stiffness with intra-articular corticosteroid injections in the hips, knees, ankles, elbows, and shoulders. She developed osteopenia and a compression fracture at T6 and hypertension treated with propranolol as well as a cushingoid appearance as complications of steroid treatment. She had persistent hepatomegaly and intermittent pleuritis as well as retrognathia and continued active arthritis in multiple joints (Fig. 1). She had restricted longitudinal growth and was started on growth hormone at age 7 years; however, her height and weight remained below the first percentile at age 12 years (Fig. 2). She started treatment with an IL-6 inhibitor (tocilizumab) at age 12 years and this was more successful in controlling her arthritis and systemic symptoms. Her steroids were able to be tapered with improvement of her cushingoid appearance and resolution of hypertension. She continued, however, to have bilateral knee flexion contractures, hip flexion contractures, and severe degenerative changes of the bilateral hips (Fig. 3). She underwent cementless right total hip arthroplasty at age 13 years by an orthopedic surgeon experienced in arthroplasty in young patients. The procedure was complicated by acute blood loss anemia requiring transfusion. She ultimately reported substantial improvement of her right hip pain. Her growth improved after steroids were stopped and she had increased to the second percentile for height and 31st percentile for weight at age 16 years (see Fig. 2). At age 19 years, her arthritis was well controlled on tocilizumab and celecoxib, and she was doing well in college.

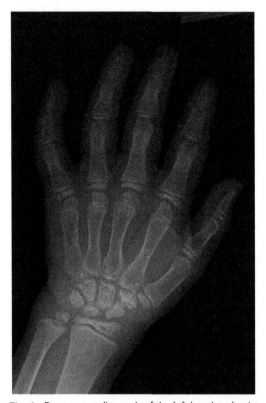

Fig. 1. Bone age radiograph of the left hand and wrist of a female patient with systemic JIA at age 9 years and 4 months. Skeletal age of 6 years and 10 months is less than her chronologic age. There is periarticular osteopenia and soft tissue swelling visible at the wrist and proximal interphalangeal joints, with sclerosis and irregularity at the carpal ossification centers and distal radial epiphysis.

is most pronounced in the morning and improves with activity.[2] Most patients with oligoarticular JIA have a remitting course; however, there is a subset of children in the extended oligoarticular group who develop involvement of 5 or more joints after the first 6 months of disease and have a course similar to patients in the RF-negative polyarthritis group.[2,4] Children with untreated unilateral knee involvement may have overgrowth of the affected limb resulting in clinically significant limb length inequality. This develops more commonly in children who present prior to age 3 years (Box 2).[16]

POLYARTHRITIS

Polyarthritis typically presents insidiously with symmetric involvement of 5 or more joints, often including large and small joints, the temporomandibular joints, and cervical spine.[4] Temporomandibular joint involvement may result in micrognathia.[2,17] Children with polyarthritis

may have systemic features, such as low-grade fevers, lymphadenopathy, and hepatosplenomegaly, but they are not as severe as in systemic-onset JIA and rash is rare.[13] Anemia of chronic disease may be present but also is less severe than in systemic-onset JIA.[18] Polyarthritis is subcategorized into patients with at least 2 positive tests for RF and those negative for RF.[1] Children with RF-positive polyarthritis tend to resemble those patients with adult rheumatoid arthritis. They often are girls older than 8 years with symmetric small joint arthritis, rheumatoid nodules, and erosive synovitis, whereas chronic uveitis is rare.[4] Hip arthritis is a poor prognostic sign in these patients and is likely to result in functional disability.[19] RF-negative polyarthritis can present at any age but is more likely to present younger than RF-positive disease with median onset at 6.5 years of age[12] and is also more common in girls, with a female-to-male ratio of 3:1 (Box 3).[4]

PSORIATIC ARTHRITIS

Psoriatic arthritis in children usually presents with asymmetric oligoarthritis or polyarthritis affecting both large and small joints. Presence of other criteria at disease onset include psoriasis in a first-degree family member (69%), pitting of the nails (67%), and dactylitis (39%).[12,20] Dactylitis is fusiform swelling or sausage digit, resulting from flexor tendon sheath inflammation.[2] The presence of psoriasis skin rash is relatively uncommon at diagnosis (13%–43%) but may develop later in the disease course.[12,20] In children younger than 5 years, a small number of affected fingers or toes may be relatively asymptomatic but result in overgrowth of the involved digits.[4] Axial arthritis may be present as well.[20,21] Median age of onset for psoriatic arthritis is 4.5 years to 10.1 years with slightly more girls than boys (1.6–2.3 times as many) affected.[12,20,22] Uveitis develops in 14% to 17% of patients.[20,21] Children with psoriatic arthritis are likely to develop polyarthritis (87%) with a relapsing and remitting course leading to irreversible joint damage.[22] Severe distal interphalangeal joint involvement and arthritis mutilans are uncommon.[4,22]

ENTHESITIS RELATED ARTHRITIS

Enthesitis-related arthritis is diagnosed in children with arthritis or enthesitis and 2 or more of the following: sacroiliac (SI) tenderness or inflammatory lumbosacral pain, HLA-B27 positive, onset of arthritis in a boy older than 6 years, symptomatic anterior uveitis, and history in a first-degree relative of ankylosing spondylitis,

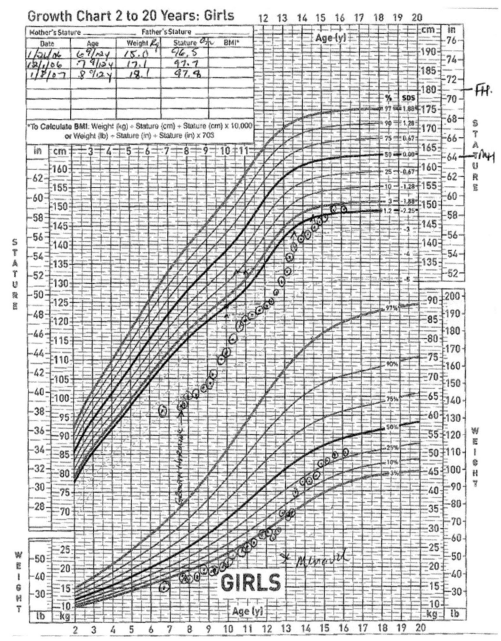

Fig. 2. Growth chart for patient with systemic JIA demonstrating significant growth restriction with height and weight well below the first percentile for age. Some increase in height is noted with growth hormone treatment. Improvement in percentile for both height and weight occurred after beginning treatment with an IL-6 inhibitor at 12 years of age. Menarche is noted at age 13 years. (*Adapted from* Centers for Disease Control and Prevention (CDC). National Center for Health Statistics. Clinical Growth Charts. Available at: https://www.cdc.gov/growth-charts/data/set1clinical/cj41l022.pdf. Accessed May 23, 2019.)

enthesitis-related arthritis, sacroiliitis with inflammatory bowel disease, Reiter syndrome, or anterior uveitis.[1] Enthesitis is demonstrated on examination by tenderness to palpation over the tibial tubercle, iliac crest, attachments of the patellar and quadriceps tendon to the patella, Achilles tendon insertion, and plantar fascia.[4] Enthesopathy of the heel at the plantar fascia and Achilles attachments is common in enthesitis-related arthritis and may be the primary site of symptoms.[23,24] Enthesitis presenting as tenderness at the Achilles insertion or

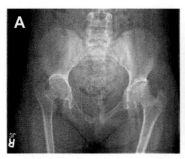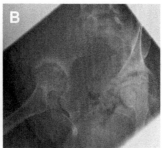

Fig. 3. (A) Anteroposterior pelvis and (B) lateral right hip radiographs at age 13 years in a patient with systemic JIA demonstrating severe degenerative changes of the bilateral hips.

inferior pole of the patella in an adolescent can easily be confused with Sever disease or Sinding-Larsen–Johansson syndrome and delay identification of an inflammatory condition. Acute

anterior uveitis can occur, typically presenting with a painful red eye and photophobia[4] and has a strong association with the presence of HLA-B27 positivity (50%) (Box 4).[25]

EXTRA-ARTICULAR MANIFESTATIONS

Uveitis affects 20% of children with JIA, most commonly those with oligoarticular arthritis.[26] Although in 50% of those affected the uveitis is effectively managed with topical medications, it is severe enough to threaten vision despite attempted treatment in 25%.[27] Therefore, routine ophthalmologic examinations with slit lamp evaluation are recommended for all children with JIA[26] because most cases are initially asymptomatic, and early detection and prompt treatment can prevent vision loss.[28] Uveitis occurs independently of the presence of joint inflammation. Many of the pharmacologic agents used to manage inflammatory arthritis are effective in control of uveitis.[29]

Nonarticular manifestations are unusual in most JIA subtypes, with the major exception of systemic juvenile arthritis. Patients with systemic disease may develop pericarditis, pleuritis, hepatitis, MAS, and profound anemia. Decades into the course of systemic disease, some individuals can develop secondary amyloidosis.[30]

ETIOLOGY

Genetic factors contribute to etiology with increased risk of JIA in patients with a strong family history of autoimmune disorders, especially psoriatic and enthesitis-related arthritis.[31] Monozygotic twins demonstrate a 25% to 40% concordance in prevalence of JIA.[31,32] There probably are several environmental and genetic factors that individually or in common lead to the development of JIA in a susceptible child. Although there is some evidence that onset of JIA can be triggered by acute infections, including parvovirus, Epstein-Barr virus, enteric

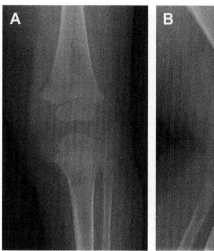 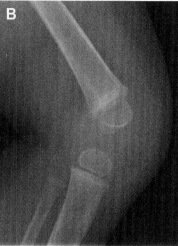

Fig. 4. (A) Anteroposterior and (B) lateral radiographs of the left knee demonstrating an effusion in a 13-month-old boy presenting with oligoarticular JIA.

bacteria, and streptococcus A, these studies involved only small numbers of JIA patients and often did not include a control group.[33] Currently, definitive knowledge of the interplay of genetic and infectious factors is not established.

An imbalance between proinflammatory and anti-inflammatory cytokines has been noted in systemic JIA, with elevated levels of proinflammatory cytokines interleukin (IL)-1, IL-6, and IL-2 shown to be involved in pathogenesis.[5,34–36] Monocytes/macrophages and neutrophils, rather than lymphocytes, are the primary cells involved.[37] Features typical of autoimmune diseases, such as associations with major histocompatibility complexes, autoantibodies, and autoreactive T-lymphocytes, are absent.[5] Therefore, systemic JIA is now being thought of as an autoinflammatory condition rather than a classic autoimmune disease.[5,37] Clinical improvement has been observed with IL-1 and IL-6 targeted therapies.[5,35,37] Tumor necrosis factor (TNF)-α inhibitors are frequently effective in treatment of other forms of JIA[38] but have been shown

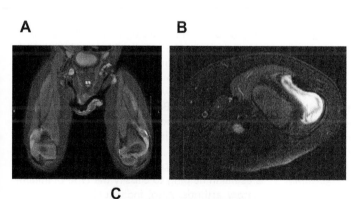

Fig. 5. (A) Coronal T2-weighted MRI of the bilateral knees and (B, C) axial T2-weighted MRI slices of the left knee demonstrating effusion and synovitis of the bilateral knees in a 13-month-old boy with oligoarticular JIA. Both B and C are axial T2-weighted MRI slices of the left knee. B is at the level of the suprapatellar pouch and C is at the level of the patella including synovitis posterior to the femoral condyles.

Box 3
Rheumatoid factor–negative polyarthritis case example

A 2-year-old girl presented with morning stiffness and swelling in multiple joints. She did not have fevers or other systemic symptoms and had no family history of any rheumatologic or autoimmune conditions. She had anemia of chronic disease and significant growth restriction. She tested negative for RF. She was treated with NSAIDs, prednisone, methotrexate, adalimumab, and abatacept but had persistently active disease. Her family had significant difficulty with regular medication administration, and following through with recommended eye examinations, laboratory tests, physical therapy and occupational therapy, and bracing. She was supported by a multidisciplinary team of physicians, social workers, dieticians, orthotists, and nurses. She continued to have micrognathia; limited mouth opening; restricted cervical spine range of motion; flexion contractures of the bilateral elbows, hips, and knees; and limited motion of the ankles and subtalar joints, with pes planovalgus deformities, hallux valgus deformities, swan neck and boutonniere deformities of several fingers. She had temporary relief from several rounds of intra-articular corticosteroid injections of the larger joints. She ultimately had better control of the arthritis with sulfasalazine and tocilizumab. At age 9 years she was 128.8 cm tall (9.9th percentile) and weighed 19.9 kg (0.1 percentile).

Box 4
Enthesitis-related arthritis case example

A 9-year-old boy presented with swelling of multiple joints. He had anemia and subsequently was diagnosed with inflammatory bowel disease. HLA-B27 tested positive. RF and ANA were negative. He had a family history of multiple paternal relatives with arthritis in their back, although no formal diagnosis of ankylosing spondylitis. He developed increasing pain and stiffness of the spine and SI joints with loss of lumbar lordosis. He was treated with NSAIDs, prednisone, hydroxychloroquine, and methotrexate. At age 14 years he continued to have active arthritis of the spine, bilateral hips, knees, ankles, and right wrist with flexion contractures of the hips and knees. He had developed dislocation of the sternum with associated pectus carinatum chest deformity (Fig. 6). He was malnourished (weight loss from 50kg at age 12 to 33.6kg at age 14 years). During evaluation for chest wall reconstruction he was found to have aortic insufficiency. He underwent a Ross procedure (pulmonary autograft aortic valve replacement and pulmonary valve replacement with pulmonary homograft) with partial repair of pectus carinatum at 15 years of age and revision pectus carinatum repair with a Ravitch procedure at age 17. He continued to have active polyarthritis but his parents were concerned about potential risks of starting a biologic agent and elected to defer this. At age 19 years he began treatment with etanercept and was able to achieve remission.

to have a fair to poor response in more than half of children with systemic JIA.[39]

EPIDEMIOLOGY

The incidence of JIA has been reported from 1.9 to 23 per 100,000.[31,40,41] Populations studied most often include whites in North America and Europe. Oligoarthritis is the most frequent type of JIA with an incidence of 3.7/100,000, followed by polyarthritis 1.6/100,000, systemic arthritis 0.6/100,000, and psoriatic arthritis 0.5/100,000.[42] Overall incidence of JIA is more common in girls (10/100,000) than boys (5.7/100,000)[42] but enthesitis-related arthritis is more common in boys.[31,43]

LABORATORY EVALUATION

Routine laboratory studies are normal in most subtypes of JIA. Indicators of inflammation (CRP, sedimentation rate, and so forth) also

can be normal, especially with involvement of only a few joints. Serologic studies positive in JIA include antinuclear antibody (ANA), which is positive in oligoarticular and polyarticular subtypes. A subgroup of polyarticular JIAs have RF and/or anti-CCP, which correlates with a worse prognosis.[44] HLA-B27 is positive in 70% to 90% of youths with psoriatic arthritis or enthesitis-related arthritis. This HLA haplotype is present in 10% of the white population overall. Screening for the presence of HLA-B27 antigen is useful in helping to classify the type of inflammatory arthritis. Also, individuals with spondyloarthropathy who have HLA-B27 are at higher risk for a more severe course.[45]

Rheumatic disorders are not diagnosed solely on the basis of laboratory results. Initial laboratory studies should be chosen based on a child's clinical history and examination and the diagnoses being considered. Wide-based screening panels for rheumatic diseases are not useful. Initial work-up should include a complete blood cell count with differential and a test for acute

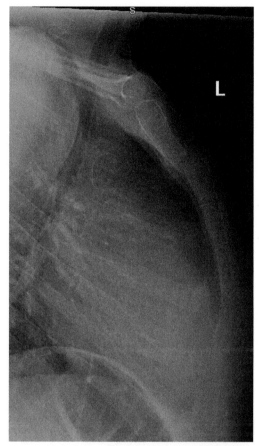

Fig. 6. Lateral sternal radiograph demonstrating anterior dislocation of the sternum from the manubrium in a 14-year-old male patient with enthesitis-related arthritis.

MANAGEMENT GOALS

Management of JIA is individualized based on the degree and site of inflammation. The goal is to minimize joint inflammation. Response to treatment is measured by a patient's joint count, laboratory indications of inflammation, and patient and practitioner assessment of joint inflammation and clinical symptoms, such as pain and morning stiffness. There are published clinical scores used in the clinic setting and in therapeutic trials that can be used to monitor disease activity. Early treatment correlates with a higher chance of remission and a reduction in long-term morbidity.[48] The treatment of patients with JIA is complex and is best managed by a multidisciplinary team, including pediatric rheumatology, ophthalmology, physical and occupational therapy, social work, nursing, and orthopedic surgery.[2] The authors recommend referral to a pediatric rheumatologist in cases of chronic inflammation persisting after 6 weeks, especially polyarthritis. Starting nonsteroidal anti-inflammatory drugs (NSAIDs) therapy and treating pain are reasonable interventions that can be started by the orthopedic surgeon while the patient is awaiting rheumatology evaluation. Acute conditions, such as toxic synovitis and

phase reactants, such as CRP and erythrocyte sedimentation rate. Other tests, such as bacterial cultures, tests for acute rheumatic fever, screening for Lyme disease, uric acid, lactate dehyrodgenase, and so forth should be considered on a case-by-case basis. ANA should not be used as a screening test for JIA. More detailed rheumatic laboratory investigation would be part of the second tier of testing and might be best left to a rheumatologist to order.[46]

Radiographs at onset can be normal or show soft tissue swelling and juxta-articular osteopenia. Extensive bony changes are not evident on routine radiographs until much later in the disease. Erosive disease is usually limited to RF-positive JIA. Ultrasonography and MRI are extremely useful in assessing the extent of inflammation and joint damage and can be quite helpful in following disease progression or remission.[47]

Table 2	
Medications for childhood arthritis	
Corticosteroids	Biologics
Prednisone	T-cell inhibitors
DMARDs	Abatacept
Methotrexate	(Orencia)
Sulfasalazine	TNF inhibitors
Hydoxychloroquine[a]	Adalimumab
(Plaquenil)	(Humira)
Leflunomide[a] (Arava)	Etanercept
NSAIDs	(Enbrel)
Celecoxib (Celebrex)	Infliximab[a]
Ibuprofen (Advil,	(Remicade)
Motrin)	IL-1 antagonists
Meloxicam (Mobic)	Canikinumab
Naproxen (Aleve,	(Ilaris)
Naprosyn)	Anakinra[a]
	(Kineret)
	Rilonacept[a]
	(Arcalyst)
	IL-6 antagonists
	Tocilizumab
	(Actemra)

All medications in the table are FDA approved for use in children unless marked "a". Those medications with "a" are used off-label.

[a] Indicated medications used off-label. Brand names included in parentheses.

postinfectious reactive arthritis (ie, parvovirus and enterovirus), can be followed by the orthopedic surgeon until the inflammatory process has completely resolved and do not typically require a rheumatology referral.

PHARMACOLOGIC STRATEGIES

Choice of agent can depend on insurance coverage and whether or not the medication is Food and Drug Administration (FDA) approved for use in children (Table 2). Most children are started on a NSAID. Aspirin used to be the mainstay in management of juvenile arthritis but other NSAIDs are safer and aspirin is now rarely used. NSAIDs control pain and inflammation. When possible, medications that are in a liquid form or only need to be dosed once per day are preferable, especially for school-aged children. Intra-articular injections of corticosteroid can provide rapid relief of joint inflammation. For patients with high disease activity, a DMARD is started a few weeks into presentation according to the 2011 American College of Rheumatology recommendations.[38] Methotrexate is the standard DMARD used by rheumatologists. Sulfasalazine and leflunomide are alternate DMARDs if methotrexate cannot be used. A biologic agent, usually an inhibitor of TNF, is added if there is an inadequate response to the nonbiologic DMARD. Commonly used TNF inhibitors (based on published experience and FDA approval) include etanercept, adalimumab and infliximab. Use of 2 different agents, inhibitors of IL-1 (canakinumab) and IL-6 (tocilizumab), have markedly improved outcomes in systemic JIA.[49] TNF inhibitors and methotrexate also are the standard medications used to manage refractory uveitis. Patients not responding to TNF inhibitors are switched to other biologic agents.[38,50–52]

NONPHARMACOLOGIC STRATEGIES

- Symptomatic care for actively inflamed joints includes rest, crutches for hip arthritis, bracing for comfort, NSAIDs, topicals, and heat packs. Activity can be resumed as tolerated.
- Physical and occupational therapy can be useful in maintaining strength and range of motion. Therapists can teach patients and families about joint protection and self-care.[2] Specific range-of-motion and weight-bearing restrictions should be avoided whenever possible and patients encouraged to keep moving to help manage their arthritis symptoms.[2,4]

- Aquatic therapy with underwater resistance exercises has been shown to increase lower extremity strength and decrease pain in patients with JIA.[53]
- Low-impact aerobic exercise, such as swimming or cycling, can decrease atrophy and increase conditioning and endurance while avoiding the increased risk of injury associated with high-impact competitive sports.[2,54]
- Exercise-based and psychological interventions have been reported to have mixed to moderate beneficial effects in improving pain, functional ability, and quality of life.[55] Both strengthening and balance/proprioception exercises were found to improve pain and lower extremity function in children with JIA.[56] Children with JIA completing Pilates exercises have shown a greater increase in both the physical and psychosocial aspects of health-related quality of life compared with those participating in conventional stretching and core stability exercises.[57]
- Modalities, such as hot paraffin, may be useful for relief of hand stiffness.[4]

Table 3 Surgical treatments in juvenile idiopathic arthritis	
Synovectomy	Short-term relief of pain and swelling.[62,63] Long-term improvement in range of motion and prevention of joint destruction have not been demonstrated.[64,65]
Soft tissue contracture release	Isolated or in conjunction with arthroplasty to address flexion contractures interfering with function[59,66,67]
Guided growth	Gradual correction of angular deformity in patients with open physes[68]
Osteotomy	Limited indications for deformity correction in skeletally mature patients
Epiphysiodesis	Appropriately timed to address limb length inequality[69,70]
Arthrodesis	Most commonly utilized for end stage arthritis in the foot and ankle[2,71]
Arthroplasty	Definitive treatment of end-stage arthritis

- Splinting of the hands and wrists or night splinting of the knees or ankles may be indicated to prevent development of contractures.[2] Serial casting or dynamic splinting may be an option for children with severe flexion contractures.[4]
- One study of children with JIA who received massage by their parents 15 minutes per day for 30 days demonstrated decreased anxiety and cortisol levels, decreased self-reported and parent-reported pain levels, decreased physician assessment of pain incidence and severity, and decreased pain-limiting activities.[58]

SURGICAL TREATMENT

Safe and successful surgical treatment of children with JIA requires coordination between a team of experts, including the pediatric orthopedic surgeon, pediatric rheumatologist, anesthesiologist, and physical therapist, knowledgeable about the specific perioperative issues in JIA.[59] Soft tissue contracture release, osteotomy, and epiphysiodesis may be useful to treat deformity and limb length inequality[60] (Table 3). Arthroplasty is the definitive treatment of symptomatic severe joint destruction but can be fraught with complications in this young and sometimes medically frail patient population.[60,61]

Preoperative evaluation

Careful preoperative evaluation for both the articular and systemic manifestations of JIA as well as the effects of medications taken for treatment of the disease is essential for anesthetic planning.[72,73] The need for preoperative laboratory testing can be determined on a case-by-case basis depending on a child's general health and risk of bleeding from a planned procedure. Routine testing includes a complete blood cell count, CRP, and comprehensive metabolic panel.[72] Patients with cardiac or pulmonary involvement should see a cardiologist and pulmonologist for optimization prior to surgery. The patient's rheumatologist should be consulted regarding management of medications in the perioperative period (Table 4).

Endotracheal intubation may be challenging due to cervical spine stiffness or instability and hypoplasia of the mandible with decreased opening of the jaw.[2] An anesthesiologist should evaluate patients for extension of the cervical spine, involvement of the temporomandibular, and cricoarytenoid joints preoperatively.[74] Temporomandibular joint arthritis can lead to

Table 4 Perioperative medication management of juvenile idiopathic arthritis patients	
NSAIDs	Hold 3 d before procedure Celecoxib can be continued NSAIDs can be given for postoperative pain
Nonbiologic DMARDs Methotrexate, sulfasalazine, hydroxychloroquine, leflunomide	Continue as prescribed until surgery Hold 1–3 d after procedure, then restart
Biologic DMARDs TNF inhibitors, IL inhibitors, B-cell and T-cell inhibitors	Schedule surgery for the end of the dosing cycle Restart when wound healing is complete, typically approximately 2 wk
Glucocorticoids Prednisone, dexamethasone, methylprednisolone, hydrocortisone	Determine if patient is at risk of adrenal suppression Continue patient's usual daily dose Stress coverage Hydrocortisone, 50 mg intravenous (or 50 mg/m^2), given at time of incision, then hydrocortisone, 25 mg intravenous, every 8 h for 24 h (50 mg/m^2 in 4 divided doses) After the 24-h intravenous hydrocortisone course, resume patient's usual corticosteroid dose

Data from Goodman SM, Springer B, Guyatt G, et al. 2017 American College of Rheumatology/American Association of hip and knee surgeons guideline for the perioperative management of antirheumatic medication in patients with rheumatic diseases undergoing elective total hip or total knee arthroplasty. J Arthroplasty 2017;32(9):2628–2638.

hypoplasia of the mandible and a high incidence of upper airway obstruction in the supine position.[75] Prior to anesthesia, radiographs, including lateral flexion and extension views of the cervical spine, should be obtained in all JIA patients with neck symptoms and in those with polyarticular disease at higher risk for cervical spine involvement regardless of symptoms.[72,76,77] Direct laryngoscopy can be avoided in favor of other intubation techniques, such as fiberoptic intubation or laryngeal mask airway in patients with evidence of instability or significantly restricted range of motion.[72,73,78] Spinal and regional anesthetic techniques are useful for lower extremity procedures and can avoid the risks associated with intubation.[73]

Perioperative medication management

The American College of Rheumatology has published standards on perioperative medication management in the rheumatic diseases.[79] Ideally, a patient's joint disease and systemic disease (if present) are in good control prior to a planned a surgical procedure. In general, there is a need to balance patient safety with the risk of precipitating a flare of disease if DMARDs are to be discontinued. Recommendations are in Table 4. NSAIDs reversibly inhibit platelet aggregation and should be held 3 days before a planned procedure. They can be restarted soon after surgery as needed for pain management. Nonbiologic DMARDs (methotrexate, sulfasalazine, hydroxychloroquine, and leflunomide) do not need to be held. There was concern in the past that methotrexate could interfere with wound healing but recent studies of continued use during the perioperative period have shown no impact on recovery. Similarly, the nonbiologic DMARDs do not have a significant impact on immune function and do not lead to an increased risk of postoperative infection. The biologic DMARDs do have a risk, however, of immune suppression and an increased risk of postoperative infection. The TNF and IL inhibitors seem to have a relatively low risk for infection, and the recommendation is to schedule the surgery at the end of the dosing period and restart when wound healing is complete, usually approximately 2 weeks postoperatively.[79,80]

Chronic glucocorticoid use increases the risk of postoperative wound infection and poor wound healing. These patients also are at risk of adrenal suppression and the need for stress corticosteroid coverage must be considered on a case-by-case basis.[81] Giving a large dose of corticosteroid for stress coverage can itself be problematic, because large doses increase the postoperative infection risks. Determination of a serum cortisol can be helpful in identifying patients with adrenal axis suppression after glucocorticoid use.[82,83] Consider stress corticosteroid administration for any patient on daily glucocorticoids for more than 3 weeks or any patient on more than prednisone (or equivalent glucocorticoid), 5 mg daily or 10 mg every other day, on a long-term basis. Glucocorticoid should be continued throughout the perioperative course. The risk of adrenal axis suppression and precipitation of an adrenal crisis probably is low. Without further studies, however, the recommendation is to give postoperative hydrocortisone to individuals on chronic glucocorticoids. The procedures discussed in this review are, in general, moderate risk, and the child should receive the usual daily dose of glucocorticoid. Stress dose recommendations for hydrocortisone are given in Table 4. Dexamethasone should not be used, due to its lack of mineralocorticoid effect.[82–84]

Orthopedic surgical treatment

Synovectomy is controversial but may be an option for treatment of a symptomatic joint before joint destruction has occurred. It is used most commonly in large joints where the greatest benefit has been reported, such as the knee.[85,86] Arthroscopic techniques can help minimize postoperative stiffness and allow for early mobilization.[87] Unfortunately, recurrence rates of synovitis after synovectomy are high (67%–100%)[87] and deteriorating results over time are frequent.[88] The long-term joint outcome is not changed by synovectomy and joint destruction is not prevented.[64,65] A trial of at least 6 months of medical therapy, including intra-articular corticosteroid injection, is indicated prior to considering treatment with synovectomy.[2]

Soft tissue releases may be considered for flexion contracture at the hip and knee, resulting in crouch and decreased ambulatory ability.[59] Initial modest correction of motion is possible, with partial recurrence of contracture common at 3 years to 5 years.[89] Night splinting for 6 months to 12 months is recommended to maintain correction in addition to postoperative physical therapy.[2,67]

Appropriately timed epiphysiodesis can address clinically significant limb length inequality[69,70]; however, predictions of growth can be challenging depending on the age of the child, type of arthritis, and success of medical treatment.[68]

Total joint arthroplasty is indicated in the adolescent with severe pain and function limiting joint destruction.[90,91] Open physes are not an absolute contraindication for total hip arthroplasty and total knee arthroplasty can be performed without resulting in growth disturbance (although all physes were closed within 2 years of arthroplasty in one series).[61,91,92] When both the hip and knee are candidates for arthroplasty, the hip typically is approached first in order to facilitate rehabilitation of the knee.[61,91] Preoperative planning must account for technical challenges related to small bone size, osteoporosis, contractures, and possible need for custom prostheses in up to 50% of patients.[61,91–93] Significant improvement in pain and function can be obtained in patients with JIA undergoing total hip arthroplasty. In 1 series, Harris hip scores improved from 34 points (range 0–65) prior to surgery to 85 points (range 33–100) postoperatively.[94] Patients with JIA undergoing total hip arthroplasty were noted to have a 26% incidence of perioperative complications with the majority being medical complications, primarily anemia. There was a 2.8% incidence of orthopedic complications comprised mostly of periprosthetic fractures thought to be related to osteopenia and difficult femoral geometry.[95] Aseptic loosening has been the primary long-term concern and a trend toward cementless implants has been occurring.[61,90–94,96,97] The 10-year implant survival for patients with JIA undergoing total hip arthroplasty before 35 years of age is 85% and was significantly longer for patients older than 25 years compared with younger than 25 years of age (89% vs 84%; $P = .04$).[98] Although less common than hip or knee arthroplasty, total elbow arthroplasty has been performed for adult patients with JIA, with 75% good to excellent results at mean 10.5-year follow-up.[99] Hemiarthroplasty in the shoulder for young adults with JIA also has been reported, with clinically meaningful decrease in pain and excellent/very good Constant-Murley scores in 43% of patients, and good/fair scores in 57% of patients with no poor outcomes at mean 10.4-year follow-up (range 5.8–13.9 years).[100]

SELF-MANAGEMENT STRATEGIES

The presence of a chronic disease like JIA is a tremendous stress to both parents and children. Stress can include psychological and physical as well as financial stresses. Both parent and child are at risk of developing mood disorders, such as depression and anxiety. Both stressors and mood disorders have an impact on the disease symptoms in children with JIA.[101] Referral for counseling, participation with support groups, attendance at family support meetings, and online peer support all can help the child and family cope.[102–104] The Arthritis Foundation and the American College of Rheumatology have several online resources for families. The Arthritis Foundation has a yearly national meeting for families and local Arthritis Foundation chapters can provide financial support for families who otherwise could not afford to attend.

EVALUATION, ADJUSTMENT, AND RECURRENCE

JIA can be a difficult condition to diagnose and is even more challenging to manage. In contrast to adult patients with rheumatic disease, children are still growing and have ongoing emotional, physical, and physiologic needs that are not present in adults. All JIA patients should be cared for by practitioners with appropriate training and experience in management of these complex disorders. The usual JIA patient is seen every 3 months by a rheumatologist and medications are adjusted accordingly based on disease activity. Routine laboratory studies are obtained to assess for disease activity and to monitor for drug side effects.[105] Most rheumatic disorders, including JIA, are characterized by remissions and clinical exacerbations. For JIA in clinical remission, medications are withdrawn 6 months to 12 months after obtaining remission. Once medications are withdrawn, a child needs to be followed regularly to assess for disease recurrence.[106–109] Musculoskeletal ultrasound is a useful tool both for following disease activity and for predicting relapse.[108] Ultrasound is widely available and noninvasive. Ultrasound can detect effusions, increased blood flow, and synovial thickening, all suggestive of active synovitis. Ultrasound also can facilitate joint injection and arthrocentesis.[46] Relapse rate varies according to JIA subtype and can range from 0% to 50%.[105–109] When a child relapses, the treating physician makes a clinical decision of whether or not the child should be trialed on a new medication or the previous medications restarted.

SUMMARY

JIA is a challenging disorder to manage. Clinical expression of disease in JIA can range from involvement of a single joint to widespread destructive arthritis, blinding uveitis, and/or overwhelming systemic inflammation, leading to death from MAS. Clinical course can be intermittent or relentlessly progressive. Medical management guided by a pediatric rheumatologist is vital to the care of patients with JIA. Regular ophthalmology examinations with slit lamp evaluation are recommended to detect uveitis. Orthopedic surgical treatment may be indicated to address deformity, limb length inequality, or end-stage arthritis. Evaluation of the cervical spine and appropriate medication management in consultation with a patient's rheumatologist are essential in perioperative care. Preoperative planning should take into account patient deformity, contracture, small size, osteopenia, and medical comorbidities. With careful perioperative coordination and planning, surgical treatment can result in significant relief of pain and functional improvement for patients with JIA.

REFERENCES

1. Petty RE, Southwood TR, Manners P, et al. International League of Associations for Rheumatology classification of juvenile idiopathic arthritis: second revision, Edmonton, 2001. J Rheumatol 2004;31(2):390–2. Available at: http://www.ncbi.nlm.nih.gov/pubmed/14760812. Accessed January 31, 2019.

2. Herring JA. Arthritis. In: Herring JA, editor. Tachdjian's pediatric orthopaedics. 5th edition. Philadelphia: Saunders; 2014. p. 1009–16. Available at: https://www-clinicalkey-com.ezproxy.med.wmich.edu/#!/content/book/3-s2.0-B9781437715491000 26X?scrollTo=%23hl0000529. Accessed January 31, 2019.

3. Cuesta IA, Kerr K, Simpson P, et al. Subspecialty referrals for pauciarticular juvenile rheumatoid arthritis. Arch Pediatr Adolesc Med 2000;154(2):122–5. Available at: http://www.ncbi.nlm.nih.gov/pubmed/10665597. Accessed February 17, 2019.

4. Wright DA. Juvenile Idiopathic Arthritis. In: Morrissy RT, Weinstein S, editors. Lovell and Winter's pediatric orthopaedics. 6th ed. Philadelphia: Lippincott Williams & Wilkins; 2006. p. 405–37.

5. Hay AD, Ilowite NT. Systemic juvenile idiopathic arthritis: a review. Pediatr Ann 2012;41(11):e232–7.

6. Goldenberg J, Ferraz MB, Pessoa AP, et al. Symptomatic cardiac involvement in juvenile rheumatoid arthritis. Int J Cardiol 1992;34(1):57–62. Available at: http://www.ncbi.nlm.nih.gov/pubmed/1548110. Accessed February 12, 2019.

7. Still GF. On a form of chronic joint disease in children. Med Chir Trans 1897;80:47–60, 9. Available at: http://www.ncbi.nlm.nih.gov/pubmed/20896907. Accessed January 31, 2019.

8. Behrens EM, Beukelman T, Gallo L, et al. Evaluation of the presentation of systemic onset juvenile rheumatoid arthritis: data from the Pennsylvania Systemic Onset Juvenile Arthritis Registry (PASOJAR). J Rheumatol 2008;35(2):343–8. Available at: http://www.ncbi.nlm.nih.gov/pubmed/18085728. Accessed February 10, 2019.

9. Schneider R, Lang BA, Reilly BJ, et al. Prognostic indicators of joint destruction in systemic-onset juvenile rheumatoid arthritis. J Pediatr 1992;120(2 Pt 1):200–5. Available at: http://www.ncbi.nlm.nih.gov/pubmed/1735815. Accessed February 12, 2019.

10. Sawhney S, Woo P, Murray KJ. Macrophage activation syndrome: a potentially fatal complication of rheumatic disorders. Arch Dis Child 2001;85(5):421–6. Available at: http://www.ncbi.nlm.nih.gov/pubmed/11668110. Accessed April 30, 2019.

11. Ruscitti P, Rago C, Breda L, et al. Macrophage activation syndrome in Still's disease: analysis of clinical characteristics and survival in paediatric and adult patients. Clin Rheumatol 2017;36(12):2839–45.

12. Symmons DP, Jones M, Osborne J, et al. Pediatric rheumatology in the United Kingdom: data from the British Pediatric Rheumatology Group National Diagnostic Register. J Rheumatol 1996;23(11):1975–80. Available at: http://www.ncbi.nlm.nih.gov/pubmed/8923378. Accessed February 17, 2019.

13. Cassidy JT, Levinson JE, Bass JC, et al. A study of classification criteria for a diagnosis of juvenile rheumatoid arthritis. Arthritis Rheum 1986;29(2):274–81. Available at: http://www.ncbi.nlm.nih.gov/pubmed/3485433. Accessed February 17, 2019.

14. Hensinger RN, DeVito PD, Ragsdale CG. Changes in the cervical spine in juvenile rheumatoid arthritis. J Bone Joint Surg Am 1986;68(2):189–98. Available at: http://www.ncbi.nlm.nih.gov/pubmed/3944157. Accessed February 17, 2019.

15. Punaro M. Rheumatologic conditions in children who may present to the orthopaedic surgeon. J Am Acad Orthop Surg 2011;19(3):163–9. Available at: http://www.ncbi.nlm.nih.gov/pubmed/21368097. Accessed February 17, 2019.

16. Vostrejs M, Hollister JR. Muscle atrophy and leg length discrepancies in pauciarticular juvenile rheumatoid arthritis. Am J Dis Child 1988;142(3):343–5. Available at: http://www.ncbi.nlm.nih.gov/pubmed/3344725. Accessed February 17, 2019.

17. Olson L, Eckerdal O, Hallonsten AL, et al. Craniomandibular function in juvenile chronic arthritis. A clinical and radiographic study. Swed Dent J 1991;15(2):71–83. Available at: http://www.ncbi.nlm.nih.gov/pubmed/2063264. Accessed February 17, 2019.

18. Peeters HR, Jongen-Lavrencic M, Raja AN, et al. Course and characteristics of anaemia in patients

with rheumatoid arthritis of recent onset. Ann Rheum Dis 1996;55(3):162–8. Available at: http://www.ncbi.nlm.nih.gov/pubmed/8712878. Accessed February 17, 2019.

19. Blane CE, Ragsdale CG, Hensinger RN. Late effects of JRA on the hip. J Pediatr Orthop 1987; 7(6):677–80. Available at: http://www.ncbi.nlm.nih.gov/pubmed/3429653. Accessed February 17, 2019.

20. Roberton DM, Cabral DA, Malleson PN, et al. Juvenile psoriatic arthritis: followup and evaluation of diagnostic criteria. J Rheumatol 1996;23(1): 166–70. Available at: http://www.ncbi.nlm.nih.gov/pubmed/8838527. Accessed February 17, 2019.

21. Southwood TR, Petty RE, Malleson PN, et al. Psoriatic arthritis in children. Arthritis Rheum 1989; 32(8):1007–13. Available at: http://www.ncbi.nlm.nih.gov/pubmed/2765001. Accessed February 17, 2019.

22. Shore A, Ansell BM. Juvenile psoriatic arthritis–an analysis of 60 cases. J Pediatr 1982;100(4):529–35. Available at: http://www.ncbi.nlm.nih.gov/pubmed/7199570. Accessed February 17, 2019.

23. Gerster JC, Piccinin P. Enthesopathy of the heels in juvenile onset seronegative B-27 positive spondyloarthropathy. J Rheumatol 1985;12(2):310–4. Available at: http://www.ncbi.nlm.nih.gov/pubmed/3875722. Accessed February 17, 2019.

24. Weiss PF, Klink AJ, Behrens EM, et al. Enthesitis in an inception cohort of enthesitis-related arthritis. Arthritis Care Res (Hoboken) 2011;63(9):1307–12.

25. Derhaag PJ, de Waal LP, Linssen A, et al. Acute anterior uveitis and HLA-B27 subtypes. Invest Ophthalmol Vis Sci 1988;29(7):1137–40. Available at: http://www.ncbi.nlm.nih.gov/pubmed/3262094. Accessed February 17, 2019.

26. American Academy of Pediatrics Section on Rheumatology and Section on Ophthalmology. Guidelines for ophthalmologic examinations in children with juvenile rheumatoid arthritis. Pediatrics 1993; 92(2):295–6. Available at: http://www.ncbi.nlm.nih.gov/pubmed/8337036. Accessed February 17, 2019.

27. Kanski JJ. Uveitis in juvenile chronic arthritis: Incidence, clinical features and prognosis. Eye 1988; 2(6):641–5.

28. Cassidy J, Kivlin J, Lindsley C, et al. Section on rheumatology, section on ophthalmology. ophthalmologic examinations in children with juvenile rheumatoid arthritis. Pediatr 2006;117(5): 1843–5.

29. Dick AD, Rosenbaum JT, Al-Dhibi HA, et al. Guidance on noncorticosteroid systemic immunomodulatory therapy in noninfectious uveitis. Ophthalmology 2018;125(5):757–73.

30. Lane T, Pinney JH, Gilbertson JA, et al. Changing epidemiology of AA amyloidosis: clinical observations over 25 years at a single national referral centre. Amyloid 2017;24(3):162–6.

31. Palman J, Shoop-Worrall S, Hyrich K, et al. Update on the epidemiology, risk factors and disease outcomes of Juvenile idiopathic arthritis. Best Pract Res Clin Rheumatol 2018;32(2): 206–22.

32. Prahalad S, Ryan MH, Shear ES, et al. Twins concordant for juvenile rheumatoid arthritis. Arthritis Rheum 2000;43(11):2611–2.

33. Rigante D, Bosco A, Esposito S. The etiology of juvenile idiopathic arthritis. Clin Rev Allergy Immunol 2015;49(2):253–61.

34. Pascual V, Allantaz F, Arce E, et al. Role of interleukin-1 (IL-1) in the pathogenesis of systemic onset juvenile idiopathic arthritis and clinical response to IL-1 blockade. J Exp Med 2005;201(9):1479–86.

35. Yokota S, Miyamae T, Imagawa T, et al. Therapeutic efficacy of humanized recombinant anti-interleukin-6 receptor antibody in children with systemic-onset juvenile idiopathic arthritis. Arthritis Rheum 2005;52(3):818–25.

36. de Benedetti F, Martini A. Targeting the interleukin-6 receptor: a new treatment for systemic juvenile idiopathic arthritis? Arthritis Rheum 2005;52(3):687–93.

37. Vastert SJ, Kuis W, Grom AA. Systemic JIA: new developments in the understanding of the pathophysiology and therapy. Best Pract Res Clin Rheumatol 2009;23(5):655–64.

38. Beukelman T, Patkar NM, Saag KG, et al. 2011 American College of Rheumatology recommendations for the treatment of juvenile idiopathic arthritis: initiation and safety monitoring of therapeutic agents for the treatment of arthritis and systemic features. Arthritis Care Res (Hoboken) 2011;63(4):465–82.

39. Kimura Y, Pinho P, Walco G, et al. Etanercept treatment in patients with refractory systemic onset juvenile rheumatoid arthritis. J Rheumatol 2005; 32(5):935–42. Available at: http://www.ncbi.nlm.nih.gov/pubmed/15868633. Accessed February 12, 2019.

40. Prieur AM, Le Gall E, Karman F, et al. Epidemiologic survey of juvenile chronic arthritis in France. Comparison of data obtained from two different regions. Clin Exp Rheumatol 1987;5(3): 217–23. Available at: http://www.ncbi.nlm.nih.gov/pubmed/3501354. Accessed February 13, 2019.

41. Savolainen E, Kaipiainen-Seppänen O, Kröger L, et al. Total incidence and distribution of inflammatory joint diseases in a defined population: results from the Kuopio 2000 arthritis survey. J Rheumatol 2003;30(11):2460–8. Available at: http://www.ncbi.nlm.nih.gov/pubmed/14677193. Accessed February 13, 2019.

42. Thierry S, Fautrel B, Lemelle I, et al. Prevalence and incidence of juvenile idiopathic arthritis: a systematic review. Joint Bone Spine 2014;81(2):112–7.

43. Gmuca S, Xiao R, Brandon TG, et al. Multicenter inception cohort of enthesitis-related arthritis: variation in disease characteristics and treatment approaches. Arthritis Res Ther 2017;19(1):84.

44. Espinosa M, Gottlieb BS. Juvenile idiopathic arthritis. Pediatr Rev 2012;33(7):303–13.

45. Berntson L, Nordal E, Aalto K, et al. HLA-B27 predicts a more chronic disease course in an 8-year followup cohort of patients with juvenile idiopathic arthritis. J Rheumatol 2013;40(5):725–31.

46. Haines KA. The approach to the child with joint complaints. Pediatr Clin North Am 2018;65(4):623–38.

47. Malattia C, Damasio MB, Magnaguagno F, et al. Magnetic resonance imaging, ultrasonography, and conventional radiography in the assessment of bone erosions in juvenile idiopathic arthritis. Arthritis Rheum 2008;59(12):1764–72.

48. Shenoi S. Juvenile idiopathic arthritis - changing times, changing terms, changing treatments. Pediatr Rev 2017;38(5):221–32.

49. Higgins GC. Complications of treatments for pediatric rheumatic diseases. Pediatr Clin North Am 2018;65(4):827–54. https://doi.org/10.1016/j.pcl.2018.04.008.

50. Ferrara G, Mastrangelo G, Barone P, et al. Methotrexate in juvenile idiopathic arthritis: advice and recommendations from the MARAJIA expert consensus meeting. Pediatr Rheumatol Online J 2018;16(1):46.

51. Jennings H, Hennessy K, Hendry GJ. The clinical effectiveness of intra-articular corticosteroids for arthritis of the lower limb in juvenile idiopathic arthritis: a systematic review. Pediatr Rheumatol Online J 2014;12(1):23.

52. Sen ES, Dick AD, Ramanan AV. Uveitis associated with juvenile idiopathic arthritis. Nat Rev Rheumatol 2015;11(6):338–48.

53. Elnaggar RK, Elshafey MA. Effects of combined resistive underwater exercises and interferential current therapy in patients with juvenile idiopathic arthritis: a randomized controlled trial. Am J Phys Med Rehabil 2016;95(2):96–102.

54. Klepper SE, Giannini MJ. Physical conditioning in children with arthritis: assessment and guidelines for exercise prescription. Arthritis Care Res 1994; 7(4):226–36. Available at: http://www.ncbi.nlm.nih.gov/pubmed/7734482. Accessed February 17, 2019.

55. Nijhof LN, Nap-van der Vlist MM, van de Putte EM, et al. Non-pharmacological options for managing chronic musculoskeletal pain in children with pediatric rheumatic disease: a systematic review. Rheumatol Int 2018. https://doi.org/10.1007/s00296-018-4136-8.

56. Baydogan SN, Tarakci E, Kasapcopur O. Effect of strengthening versus balance-proprioceptive exercises on lower extremity function in patients with juvenile idiopathic arthritis: a randomized, single-blind clinical trial. Am J Phys Med Rehabil 2015;94(6):417–24 [quiz 425-428].

57. Mendonça TM, Terreri MT, Silva CH, et al. Effects of pilates exercises on health-related quality of life in individuals with juvenile idiopathic arthritis. Arch Phys Med Rehabil 2013;94(11): 2093–102.

58. Field T, Hernandez-Reif M, Seligman S, et al. Juvenile rheumatoid arthritis: benefits from massage therapy. J Pediatr Psychol 1997;22(5):607–17. Available at: http://www.ncbi.nlm.nih.gov/pubmed/9383925. Accessed February 17, 2019.

59. Swann M. The surgery of juvenile chronic arthritis. An overview. Clin Orthop Relat Res 1990;259: 70–5. Available at: http://www.ncbi.nlm.nih.gov/pubmed/2208876. Accessed February 18, 2019.

60. Iesaka K, Kubiak EN, Bong MR, et al. Orthopedic surgical management of hip and knee involvement in patients with juvenile rheumatoid arthritis. Am J Orthop (Belle Mead NJ) 2006;35(2):67–73. Available at: http://www.ncbi.nlm.nih.gov/pubmed/16584079. Accessed February 18, 2019.

61. Abdel MP, Figgie MP. Surgical Management of the Juvenile Idiopathic Arthritis Patient with Multiple Joint Involvement. Orthop Clin North Am 2014;45(4):435–42.

62. Carl H-D, Schraml A, Swoboda B, et al. Synovectomy of the hip in patients with juvenile rheumatoid arthritis. J Bone Joint Surg Am 2007;89(9): 1986.

63. Mäenpää H, Kuusela P, Lehtinen J, et al. Elbow synovectomy on patients with juvenile rheumatoid arthritis. Clin Orthop Relat Res 2003;412(412): 65–70.

64. Jacobsen ST, Levinson JE, Crawford AH. Late results of synovectomy in juvenile rheumatoid arthritis. J Bone Joint Surg Am 1985;67(1):8–15. Available at: http://www.ncbi.nlm.nih.gov/pubmed/3968106. Accessed February 18, 2019.

65. Kvien TK, Pahle JA, Høyeraal HM, et al. Comparison of synovectomy and no synovectomy in patients with juvenile rheumatoid arthritis. A 24-month controlled study. Scand J Rheumatol 1987;16(2): 81–91. Available at: http://www.ncbi.nlm.nih.gov/pubmed/3299684. Accessed February 18, 2019.

66. Swann M, Ansell BM. Soft-tissue release of the hips in children with juvenile chronic arthritis. J Bone Joint Surg Br 1986;68(3):404–8. Available at: http://www.ncbi.nlm.nih.gov/pubmed/3733806. Accessed February 18, 2019.

67. Clarke DW, Ansell BM, Swann M. Soft-tissue release of the knee in children with juvenile chronic arthritis. J Bone Joint Surg Br 1988;70(2):

224–7. Available at: http://www.ncbi.nlm.nih.gov/pubmed/3346293. Accessed February 18, 2019.

68. Rydholm U, Brattström H, Bylander B, et al. Stapling of the knee in juvenile chronic arthritis. J Pediatr Orthop 1987;7(1):63–8. Available at: http://www.ncbi.nlm.nih.gov/pubmed/3793914. Accessed February 18, 2019.

69. Simon S, Whiffen J, Shapiro F. Leg-length discrepancies in monoarticular and pauciarticular juvenile rheumatoid arthritis. J Bone Joint Surg Am 1981; 63(2):209–15. Available at: http://www.ncbi.nlm.nih.gov/pubmed/7462277. Accessed February 18, 2019.

70. Skyttä E, Savolainen A, Kautiainen H, et al. Treatment of leg length discrepancy with temporary epiphyseal stapling in children with juvenile idiopathic arthritis during 1957-99. J Pediatr Orthop 2003;23(3): 378–80. Available at: http://www.ncbi.nlm.nih.gov/pubmed/12724604. Accessed February 18, 2019.

71. Sammarco GJ, Tablante EB. Subtalar arthrodesis. Clin Orthop Relat Res 1998;349:73–80. Available at: http://www.ncbi.nlm.nih.gov/pubmed/9584369. Accessed February 18, 2019.

72. Vieira EM, Goodman S, Tanaka PP. Anesthesia and rheumatoid arthritis. Braz J Anesthesiol 2011;61(3):367–75.

73. Lisowska B, Rutkowska-Sak L, Maldyk P, et al. Anaesthesiological problems in patients with rheumatoid arthritis undergoing orthopaedic surgeries. Clin Rheumatol 2008;27(5):553–6.

74. Skues MA, Welchew EA. Anaesthesia and rheumatoid arthritis. Anaesthesia 1993;48(11):989–97. Available at: http://www.ncbi.nlm.nih.gov/pubmed/8250199. Accessed February 23, 2019.

75. Reginster JY, Damas P, Franchimont P. Anaesthetic risks in osteoarticular disorders. Clin Rheumatol 1985;4(1):30–8. Available at: http://www.ncbi.nlm.nih.gov/pubmed/3886270. Accessed February 23, 2019.

76. Elhai M, Wipff J, Bazeli R, et al. Radiological cervical spine involvement in young adults with polyarticular juvenile idiopathic arthritis. Rheumatology 2013;52(2):267–75.

77. Hospach T, Maier J, Müller-Abt P, et al. Cervical spine involvement in patients with juvenile idiopathic arthritis - MRI follow-up study. Pediatr Rheumatol Online J 2014;12(1):9.

78. Fulling PD, Roberts JT. Fiberoptic intubation. Int Anesthesiol Clin 2000;38(3):189–217. Available at: http://www.ncbi.nlm.nih.gov/pubmed/10984853. Accessed February 24, 2019.

79. Goodman SM, Springer B, Guyatt G, et al. 2017 American College of Rheumatology/American Association of hip and knee surgeons guideline for the perioperative management of antirheumatic medication in patients with rheumatic diseases undergoing elective total hip or total

knee arthroplasty. J Arthroplasty 2017;32(9): 2628–38. https://doi.org/10.1016/j.arth.2017.05.001.

80. Axford JS, Schmerling RH, Jones SB. Preoperative evaluation and perioperative management of patients with rheumatic diseases. UpToDate; 2018.

81. Kehlet H. A rational approach to dosage and preparation of parenteral glucocorticoid substitution therapy during surgical procedures. A short review. Acta Anaesthesiol Scand 1975;19(4): 260–4. Available at: http://www.ncbi.nlm.nih.gov/pubmed/1189879. Accessed February 24, 2019.

82. Younes AK, Younes NK. Recovery of steroid induced adrenal insufficiency. Transl Pediatr 2017;6(4):269–73.

83. Liu MM, Reidy AB, Saatee S, et al. Perioperative steroid management: approaches based on current evidence. Anesthesiology 2017;127(1): 166–72.

84. Jack J, Young SB, Cooke D. Endocrinology. In: Hughes HK, Kahl L, editors. Harriet Lane Handbook. 21st edition. Amsterdam: Elsevier, Inc; 2018. p. 255–89.

85. Rydholm U, Elborgh R, Ranstam J, et al. Synovectomy of the knee in juvenile chronic arthritis. A retrospective, consecutive follow-up study. J Bone Joint Surg Br 1986;68(2):223–8. Available at: http://www.ncbi.nlm.nih.gov/pubmed/3958007. Accessed February 18, 2019.

86. Kampner SL, Ferguson AB. Efficacy of synovectomy in juvenile rheumatoid arthritis. Clin Orthop Relat Res 1972;88:94–109. Available at: http://www.ncbi.nlm.nih.gov/pubmed/5086588. Accessed February 18, 2019.

87. Dell'Era L, Facchini R, Corona F. Knee synovectomy in children with juvenile idiopathic arthritis. J Pediatr Orthop B 2008;17(3):128–30.

88. Ovregard T, Høyeraal HM, Pahle JA, et al. A three-year retrospective study of synovectomies in children. Clin Orthop Relat Res 1990;259:76–82. Available at: http://www.ncbi.nlm.nih.gov/pubmed/2208877. Accessed February 18, 2019.

89. Witt JD, McCullough CJ. Anterior soft-tissue release of the hip in juvenile chronic arthritis. J Bone Joint Surg Br 1994;76(2):267–70. Available at: http://www.ncbi.nlm.nih.gov/pubmed/8113289. Accessed February 18, 2019.

90. Parvizi J, Lajam CM, Trousdale RT, et al. Total knee arthroplasty in young patients with juvenile rheumatoid arthritis. J Bone Joint Surg Am 2003;85-A(6):1090–4. Available at: http://www.ncbi.nlm.nih.gov/pubmed/12784008. Accessed February 18, 2019.

91. Scott RD. Total hip and knee arthroplasty in juvenile rheumatoid arthritis. Clin Orthop Relat Res 1990; 259:83–91. Available at: http://www.ncbi.nlm.nih.

gov/pubmed/2208878. Accessed February 18, 2019.

92. Sarokhan AJ, Scott RD, Thomas WH, et al. Total knee arthroplasty in juvenile rheumatoid arthritis. J Bone Joint Surg Am 1983;65(8):1071–80. Available at: http://www.ncbi.nlm.nih.gov/pubmed/6630251. Accessed February 18, 2019.

93. Haber D, Goodman SB. Total hip arthroplasty in juvenile chronic arthritis: a consecutive series. J Arthroplasty 1998;13(3):259–65. Available at: http://www.ncbi.nlm.nih.gov/pubmed/9590636. Accessed February 18, 2019.

94. Rahimtoola ZO, Finger S, Imrie S, et al. Outcome of total hip arthroplasty in small-proportioned patients. J Arthroplasty 2000;15(1):27–34. Available at: http://www.ncbi.nlm.nih.gov/pubmed/10654459. Accessed February 18, 2019.

95. Schnaser EA, Browne JA, Padgett DE, et al. Perioperative complications in patients with inflammatory arthropathy undergoing total hip arthroplasty. J Arthroplasty 2016;31(10):2286–90.

96. Carmichael E, Chaplin DM. Total knee arthroplasty in juvenile rheumatoid arthritis. A seven-year follow-up study. Clin Orthop Relat Res 1986;210:192–200. Available at: http://www.ncbi.nlm.nih.gov/pubmed/3757362. Accessed February 18, 2019.

97. Cage DJ, Granberry WM, Tullos HS. Long-term results of total arthroplasty in adolescents with debilitating polyarthropathy. Clin Orthop Relat Res 1992;283:156–62. Available at: http://www.ncbi.nlm.nih.gov/pubmed/1395240. Accessed February 18, 2019.

98. Swarup I, Lee Y, Christoph EI, et al. Implant survival and patient-reported outcomes after total hip arthroplasty in young patients with juvenile idiopathic arthritis. J Arthroplasty 2015;30(3):398–402.

99. Baghdadi YMK, Jacobson JA, Duquin TR, et al. The outcome of total elbow arthroplasty in juvenile idiopathic arthritis (juvenile rheumatoid arthritis) patients. J Shoulder Elbow Surg 2014;23(9):1374–80.

100. Ibrahim EF, Rashid A, Thomas M. Resurfacing hemiarthroplasty of the shoulder for patients with juvenile idiopathic arthritis. J Shoulder Elbow Surg 2018;27(8):1468–74.

101. Schanberg LE, Gil KM, Anthony KK, et al. Pain, stiffness, and fatigue in juvenile polyarticular arthritis: contemporaneous stressful events and mood as predictors. Arthritis Rheum 2005;52(4):1196–204.

102. Stinson J, Ahola Kohut S, Forgeron P, et al. The iPeer2-Peer Program: a pilot randomized controlled trial in adolescents with Juvenile Idiopathic Arthritis. Pediatr Rheumatol Online J 2016;14(1):48.

103. Yuwen W, Lewis FM, Walker AJ, et al. Struggling in the dark to help my child: parents' experience in caring for a young child with juvenile idiopathic arthritis. J Pediatr Nurs 2017;37:e23–9.

104. Vuorimaa H, Tamm K, Honkanen V, et al. Pain in juvenile idiopathic arthritis—a family matter. Child Heal Care 2011;40(1):34–52.

105. Giancane G, Consolaro A, Lanni S, et al. Juvenile idiopathic arthritis: diagnosis and treatment. Rheumatol Ther 2016;3(2):187–207.

106. Horton DB, Onel KB, Beukelman T, et al. Attitudes and approaches for withdrawing drugs for children with clinically inactive nonsystemic JIA: a survey of the childhood arthritis and rheumatology research alliance. J Rheumatol 2017;44(3):352–60.

107. Baszis K, Garbutt J, Toib D, et al. Clinical outcomes after withdrawal of anti-tumor necrosis factor α therapy in patients with juvenile idiopathic arthritis: a twelve-year experience. Arthritis Rheum 2011;63(10):3163–8.

108. Gremese E, Fedele AL, Alivernini S, et al. Ultrasound assessment as predictor of disease relapse in children and adults with arthritis in clinical stable remission: new findings but still unmet needs. Ann Rheum Dis 2018;77(10):1391–3.

109. Foell D, Frosch M, Schulze zur Wiesch A, et al. Methotrexate treatment in juvenile idiopathic arthritis: when is the right time to stop? Ann Rheum Dis 2004;63(2):206–8. Available at: http://www.ncbi.nlm.nih.gov/pubmed/14722212. Accessed February 24, 2019.

Hand and Wrist

Arthritis of the Thumb Interphalangeal and Finger Distal Interphalangeal Joint

John C. Wu, MD*, James H. Calandruccio, MD,
William Jacob Weller, MD, Peter R. Henning, MD,
Colin W. Swigler, MD

KEYWORDS
• Distal interphalangeal joint • Arthritis • Arthrodesis • Arthroplasty • Mucous cyst

KEY POINTS
• The interphalangeal joints are subjected to the highest joint forces in the hand. • At least 60% of individuals older than age 60 years have distal interphalangeal (DIP) joint arthritis, but not all experience symptoms. • Physiologically younger and healthier patients put higher loads on the joint for a longer time than do older, less healthy patients. These increased loads increase the risk of implant failure, making arthrodesis an attractive option, especially in young, active patients. • Interphalangeal arthrodesis has high fusion rates, with few complications, regardless of the method of fixation.

Osteoarthritis (OA) commonly affects the finger distal interphalangeal (DIP) or the thumb interphalangeal (IP) joints, which are subjected to high joint reactive forces and undergo more wear and tear than other joints in the hand. It is estimated that at least 60% of individuals older than age 60 years have DIP joint arthritis, but not all experience symptoms.[1-3] In the early stages, the joints may be painful and swollen despite normal radiographs. As the arthritis progresses, osteophytes and mucous cysts may develop; bony prominences (Heberden nodes) and angular deformities in both the coronal and sagittal planes may also develop. In the final stages, DIP joint motion may be severely restricted, making common household tasks such as opening containers, writing, and manipulating small objects, difficult or impossible. Physical examination should include the appearance of joints and overlying skin, active and passive range of motion of the affected joints,

stability, grip and pinch strength, and sensibility. Adjacent joints also should be examined because chronic DIP OA resulting in a flexion deformity can cause a secondary hyperextension deformity of the proximal interphalangeal (PIP) joint that may be more disabling than the DIP deformity. The thumb IP joint degeneration similarly may manifest early with pain and mucous cysts and later with angular and rotary defects. Radiographs typically show joint space narrowing, osteophytes, bone cysts, and sclerosis of the subchondral bone.

MUCOUS CYSTS

Mucous cysts are ganglion cysts that arise from an osteoarthritic DIP joint. They typically are painless and often present on one side of the extensor tendon, between the extensor tendon and the adjacent collateral ligament. Occasionally, the mucous cyst can compress the nail's

Disclosure Statement: The authors have nothing to disclose.
Department of Orthopaedic Surgery and Biomedical Engineering, University of Tennessee-Campbell Clinic, 1211 Union Avenue, Suite 510, Memphis, TN 38104, USA
* Corresponding author.
E-mail address: john.cheeon.wu@gmail.com

germinal matrix, causing ridging, a longitudinal groove in the nail (**Fig. 1**). If the cyst continues to enlarge, more severe nail deformities can occur with further compression.[4] Concave nail plate deformities secondary to ganglion (mucous) cyst compression of the germinal matrix are frequent. Given the subcutaneous location of the cyst, the overlying skin can become attenuated and the cyst can spontaneously drain. There is a possibility that a mucous cyst can result in a draining sinus, and infection of the finger can present in varying degrees of severity:cellulitis, soft-tissue abscess, or a septic DIP joint.[5] Patients should be counseled to avoid the temptation to puncture the cyst using nonsterile and/or ablation or cautery techniques because they usually are ineffective and increase the risk of infection.

Treatment of Mucous Cysts

In general, mucous cysts may not require treatment if there is no significant pain or signs of infection. Some cysts spontaneously resolve and others may be associated with well-tolerated nailplate deformities. Aspiration followed by steroid injection and compression wrap is a reasonable treatment option for cysts that fail to spontaneously resolve, and this can be done in the office setting.[6,7] Multiple passes are made through the cyst to facilitate decompression, and some advocate passing the needle through the joint capsule in an attempt to disrupt the source.[8] Open surgical treatment is indicated for most cysts, especially those that recur after aspiration and injection or in the presence of suspected infection. Some patients may opt to forego aspiration and injection given the higher possibility of recurrence compared with surgical excision.[8]

Surgical Considerations

The surgical approach is similar to that used for IP or DIP fusion (**Fig. 2**), with the exception that the extensor tendon should be left intact and protected throughout the procedure. The overlying skin can be excised through an elliptical incision or carefully elevated off the cyst (**Fig. 3**). The cyst is excised, along with a small portion of the joint capsule and any soft tissue between the extensor tendon and the adjacent collateral ligament. The other side of the extensor tendon can be exposed in a similar manner to expose the entire DIP joint to ensure adequate osteophyte excision, because a cyst emerging from one side of a digit may be from a lesion on the opposite side. Care should be taken not to disrupt the germinal matrix to avoid iatrogenic postoperative nail deformities.

With the DIP joint held in hyperextension, the terminal extensor tendon is carefully elevated off the phalanx proximally for protection, while preserving its distal insertion (**Fig. 4**). Removal of all surrounding osteophytes is imperative to minimize recurrence; however, excision of the cyst sac itself may not be necessary, especially if it risks violation of the germinal matrix.[9,10] Some osteophytes may have a higher chondral composition and are not always appreciated on plain

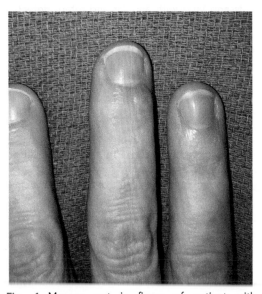

Fig. 1. Mucous cyst in finger of patient with osteoarthritis.

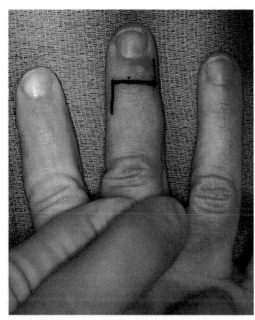

Fig. 2. Surgical approach for cyst excision.

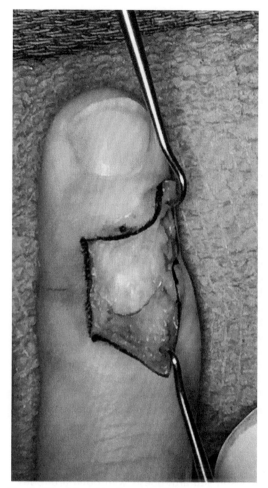

Fig. 3. Overlying skin elevated off the cyst.

radiographs, but are easily seen during surgery. A rotation flap or skin graft can be used if the wound cannot be primarily closed, although this is rarely required.[8]

Outcomes and Complications

Recurrence rates have been reported to range from 50% to 100% after aspiration and injection.[6–8] Surgical procedures that include cyst removal, partial capsulectomy, and osteophyte excision are highly successful and have much lower recurrence rates. Eaton and colleagues[9] reported 1 recurrence in a series of 44 digits, Kleinert and colleagues[11] had no recurrences in 36 cases, Fritz and colleagues[12] reported a 3% recurrence rate (JHS 1997;22B), and Rizzo and Beckenbaugh[8] reported no recurrences in 83 digits (including 29 cysts that failed to respond to aspiration and injection) with a minimum follow-up of 2 years.

Nail ridging usually resolves after joint debridement and cyst decompression. Fritz

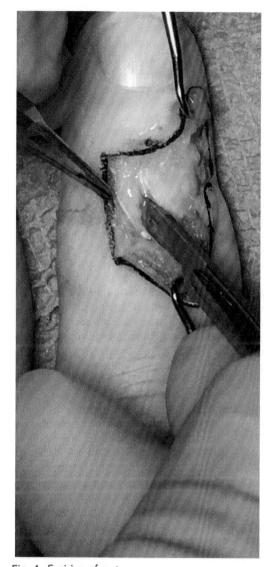

Fig. 4. Excision of cyst.

and colleagues[12] reported a 60% resolution rate of nail ridging, Kasdan and colleagues[13] had a 90% resolution, and Rizzo and Beckenbaugh[8] reported an 80% resolution rate after surgical removal. None of these studies identified factors that could increase the likelihood of persistent deformity.

Complications such as stiffness of the DIP joint, infection, persistent nail deformity, swelling, and pain appear to occur at equal rates, regardless of whether surgery or aspiration and injection is performed.[8,12] Infection rates generally are low and infection usually are superficial, such that they can be treated with oral antibiotics.[8] Infection rates are reported to be as low as 2% with needle procedures,[6,8] and between 2% and 3% for surgical procedures.[12,13] Stiffness, pain, and swelling rates ranged from 9% to 14%.[8,12,13] With the exception of infection, these complications appear to be relatively well tolerated and do not compromise clinical results.[8] Iatrogenic nail deformity is a complication that is more commonly associated with surgery and has been reported as a 7% risk in 1 study[12] and 0% in another.[8]

DISTAL INTERPHALANGEAL JOINT ARTHRODESIS

Although the appearance of the hand may be a primary patient concern, operative treatment generally should not be undertaken for strictly cosmetic reasons, but for DIP and IP deformities that interfere with hand function or severely limit motion. The functional impact of the terminal joint arthritis should be clearly defined, because sometimes quite marked visual deformities and underlying radiographic changes are associated with little functional impairment. In addition to risks and benefits of the procedure, patient expectations, handedness, occupation, and avocational activities should be discussed before surgery. Physiologically younger and healthier patients put higher loads on the joint for a longer time than do older, less healthy patients. These increased loads increase the risk of implant failure, making joint debridements and arthrodeses attractive options, especially in young, active patients. Preoperative splinting in the desired fusion position can confirm the patient's satisfaction with the position before the procedure is performed. DIP and IP joint arthroplasties are associated with substantially higher failure rates than is fusion because of the small bone dimensions and high forces across the joint; it rarely is performed. Terminal joint fusions are well tolerated and are extremely durable.

Surgical Considerations
Exposure
Surgical approaches to the DIP and IP joints include a curved dorsal incision in line with the skin creases, a dorsal H-type incision with the transverse portion parallel to the skin crease, and a transverse skin incision centered over the terminal joint with contralateral proximal and distal longitudinal extensions. When fusions are to be done, the terminal slip of the extensor tendon is transected just proximal to the joint, and the distally based terminal slip is left attached to the dorsal lip of the distal phalanx. The terminal slip is dissected sharply over the distal phalanx dorsal rim; this exposes an often elongated rim for resection and also protects the germinal matrix. The collateral ligaments are released from the neck of the middle phalanx of the fingers or the thumb proximal phalanx, allowing the joint to hyperflex to expose the entire mating surfaces of the degenerative joint.

Bone preparation
Articular cartilage and subchondral bone are removed until healthy cancellous bone is exposed. A prominent and elongated dorsal articular rim, as well as any protruding osteophytes (especially on the finger middle phalanx or thumb proximal phalanx dorsal head), should be removed. A small rongeur is ideal for this purpose. Exposure of cancellous bone is required on the mating surfaces to be fused, and sometimes the wear pattern on significantly angled DIP joints requires contouring to angles other than 90° for maximal cancellous contact with collinear middle-distal phalanx alignment. A cup-and-cone configuration is the most commonly used, although some surgeons use flat, angled surface cuts at the fusion site. Regardless of the method chosen for fusion, it is imperative to resect any soft tissue that may be interposed in the fusion site. Thus, redundant capsular tissue and collateral ligaments often are excised for both exposure and bone apposition.

Renfree[14] compared the results of percutaneous in situ arthrodesis with open arthrodesis of the DIP joint, and found that solid fusion occurred in 10 of 17 with percutaneous in situ arthrodesis compared with 11 of 12 with open arthrodesis. He concluded that open arthrodesis is better because it allows osteophyte removal and better correction of angular deformity in the coronal plane.

Method of fixation
DIP joint fusion rates are high with most fixation devices (Table 1). The technically simplest fixation is achieved with crossed Kirschner wires, which are left in to maintain the desired angular and rotational position until fusion is achieved. The wires usually are left buried, although a percutaneous method can be used. Headless screws are a popular fixation method and are associated with high fusion rates and less frequent device irritation (Fig. 5). Dickson and colleagues[15] compared Kirschner wires, cerclage wires, and headless screws and found no difference in infection rates, but higher fusion rates with headless screws. More recently, shape-memory (nitinol) staples have been reported to

Table 1
Advantages and disadvantages of fixation methods for DIP arthrodesis

Fixation Method	Advantages	Disadvantages
Kirschner wires	High fusion rate (92%–100%)	Risk of pin track infection
Interosseous wires	High fusion rate (88%–100%)	Implant prominence, may require second procedure for removal
Headless compression screws	High fusion rate (85%–100%) Stability across fusion site, no implant prominence	Difficulty in obtaining fusion in flexion, size mismatch between bone and screw, increased cost, possible nail deformity, screw cutout, screw breakage, retained implant
Headed screws	High fusion rate (95%–100%)	Prominent screw heads
Nitinol implant (X-fuse)	High fusion rate (89%–95%), allow 35° of flexion	Cost

obtain high fusion rates with few complications, with an advantage over screws of allowing 35° of flexion when desired; these devices, however, are more expensive than other fixation methods and are not intramedullary and risk causing nail matrix damage. Auzias and colleagues[16] described the use of a titanium intramedullary implant (Lync, Novastep) that is, available in straight or bent configurations, does not require removal, and can be inserted without fingertip incisions. Twenty (91%) of 22 joints were fused at latest follow-up (15 months), 18 (82%) within 3 months, and pain and function were improved. The authors cited less bulk and no need for removal as advantages of this device.

Position of fusion
Ideally, the natural cascade of the hand should be preserved to present the most aesthetically pleasing outcome. The natural cascade can be calculated on the basis of the position of the resting index finger. The index MP joint is generally positioned in 25° of flexion, and the index PIP joint is generally positioned in 40° of flexion. Flexion of the MP and PIP joints progresses in a radial-to-ulnar direction by approximately 5° per digit. Flexion of the DIP joints remains relatively constant at approximately 5°. Comparing the flexion of the joints with that of the opposite hand or with the ipsilateral hand (if the other joints are well preserved) can help guide the fusion position. Although appearance is

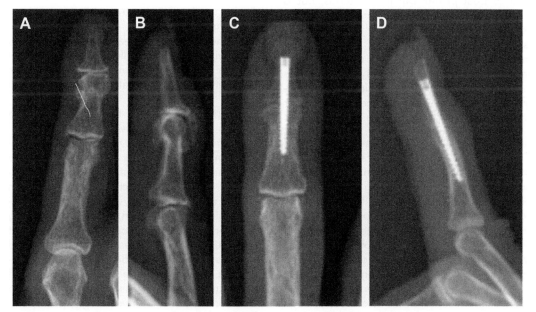

Fig. 5. (*A, B*) Osteoarthritis of the distal interphalangeal joint. (*C, D*) After fusion with a headless screw.

important, the primary concern should be function. Patients who desire a higher degree of dexterity, such as musicians, some athletes, and workers with various tools, may prefer a slightly more flexed position. The increasing use of digital devices has added another layer to the controversy over fusion position. Melamed and colleagues[17] evaluated dexterity and grip strength in 46 subjects after simulated DIP joint fusion. Index finger dexterity scores were improved when the DIP joint was splinted in 20° compared with full extension. Positioning the middle finger DIP joint in either extension or 20° of flexion did not significantly affect grip strength and dexterity; however, positioning the DIP joint in 20° of flexion may improve grip strength and dexterity over positioning it in neutral.

Outcomes and complications

Regardless of the fixation method used, fusion rates ranging from 85% to 100% have been reported with DIP arthrodesis (see Table 1). In their systematic review, Dickson and colleagues[15] reported a 96% fusion rate in 492 arthrodeses with screw fixation and a 92% fusion rate in 389 arthrodeses with K-wire fixation. Complications are infrequent (approximately 2% in most studies) and include primarily infection, skin necrosis, and implant problems (prominent screw, screw cutout, broken screw).

IMPLANT ARTHROPLASTY

DIP joint implant arthroplasty is less commonly used to treat painful DIP joint arthritis, but is a viable option when maintaining motion is desired, such as in musicians.[18] The technique uses small silicone implants that can be implanted into any digit, but it is important to protect the collateral ligaments when the procedure is done on the index digit to avoid postoperative instability from the large ulnar deviating forces from the thumb during pinch.[19]

Technique: Implant Arthroplasty

A variety of dorsal incisions can be used to expose the DIP joint. Variations in technique include preserving or dividing the extensor tendon just proximal to the DIP joint to allow extended exposure. Hyperflexion of the distal phalanx also can aid in visualization when the extensor tendon is divided. Extensor tendon preservation requires elevation of the collateral ligaments from the distal phalanx and removal of all soft tissue lateral to the extensor tendon. The DIP joint can then be accessed through these lateral windows with lateral flexion of the

distal phalanx.[19] Careful manipulation and traction should be performed to avoid intraoperative extensor tendon rupture. The middle and distal phalanx bony surfaces are prepared using an oscillating saw or rongeur. The intramedullary canal can be prepared with a small power burr or hand-held reamers. Trial implants are used to determine the appropriate size required to optimize motion and stability. After the definitive prosthesis is implanted, the extensor tendon is repaired using nonabsorbable suture if divided during exposure. Kirschner wire fixation has been described to stabilize the DIP joint in extension at the conclusion of the procedure. The technique, as described in multiple articles, requires a Kirschner wire to be inserted in a retrograde fashion through the distal phalanx into the volar portion of the flexor tendon sheath, just proximal to the DIP joint, while avoiding the implant.[20–22] Understandably, this technique is not always adopted, and extension postoperative splinting can also be done.[19,23]

Outcomes of Implant Arthroplasty

Snow and colleagues[24] reported good results with pain relief and maintenance of 40° to 45° of active motion in 7 digits. Brown[23] reported high patient satisfaction, with all 21 patients reporting complete pain relief at an average follow-up of 26 months. There was an average active range of motion of 30°, which was 9° less than preoperative values. Extensor lag was not considered a complication in this series and the average postoperative extensor lag was 12°. In this study, the extensor tendon was divided and postoperative splinting without K-wire fixation was used.

Zimmerman and colleagues[21] reported 38 digits with an average follow-up of 6 years. All patients reported decreased pain and the average active postoperative range of motion was 33° with an average extension lag of 13°. This series also divided the extensor tendon but also used postoperative K-wire fixation.[20–22]

The most recent review reported 131 replacements in 85 patients with an average follow-up of 3 years.[19] This study had 2 groups representing the different approaches, extensor tendon division and preservation, and found no statistical difference between groups regarding extensor lag, range of motion, or improvement of pain. Their other results also supported previous literature regarding reliable improvement in pain and maintaining active range of motion (mean of 39°). The mean postoperative extensor lag was 11°. Interestingly, postoperative extensor lag was observed in most digits, regardless of preservation or division of the extensor tendon. This could be due to the chronic attenuation of the terminal tendon secondary to dorsal osteophytes, with their removal causing postoperative laxity and extensor lag, or from shortening of the distal digit where the length of bone resected is more than the length provided by the implant.

Complications of Silicone Implant Arthroplasty

Brown and colleagues[23] reported 1 (5%) complication in 21 digits, a perforation of the implant through the dorsal cortex of the distal phalanx, leading to infection. Zimmerman and colleagues[21] reported 3 (10%) complications in 31 digits that required implant removal; 1 patient had an implant that eroded through the skin, another had a presumed infection, and one had persistent joint instability that eventually resulted in a phalangeal fracture. Sierakowski and colleagues[19] reported a 5% complication rate in 131 digits, with complications including superficial infection, osteomyelitis, persistent mallet deformity, lateral instability, and inadequate osteophyte resection. Fusion was the most common treatment of a failed DIP joint implant arthroplasty in all of these studies.

OTHER ARTHROPLASTY OPTIONS

When treating a painful mobile arthritic DIP joint, alternative techniques can provide pain relief while preserving range of motion and avoiding potential complications associated with implant arthroplasty. Volar plate advancement arthroplasty along with K-wire fixation can be an effective surgical treatment of posttraumatic DIP joint arthritis.[25] This technique is more commonly described for posttraumatic arthritic changes after chronic dorsal fracture-dislocation injuries of the PIP joint, but good results were reported in a series of 10 digits, with minimal to no pain and preserved average active range of motion of 42°.[25] Interpositional arthroplasty, using a free extensor retinaculum or palmaris longus tendon graft, also has been described for symptomatic arthritic DIP joint with good results in a small series of 5 digits.[26] Another surgical option with reported successful results is open cheilectomy and debridement.[27]

SUMMARY

The IP and DIP joints are subjected to the highest joint forces in the hand, and at least 60% of individuals older than age 60 years have DIP joint arthritis. Regardless of the fixation method,

DIP fusion has high success rates, is well tolerated, and is extremely durable, making it an attractive option for younger, active patients. Less active and older patients are also well served by DIP fusion, which yields stability and increases strength required for normal daily living activities.

REFERENCES

1. Dahaghin S, Bierma-Zeinstra SM, Ginai AZ, et al. Prevalence and pattern of radiographic hand osteoarthritis and association with pain and disability (the Rotterdam study). Ann Rheum Dis 2005;64:682–7.
2. Kalichman L, Cohen Z, Kobyliansky E, et al. Patterns of joint distribution in hand osteoarthritis: contribution of age, sex, and handedness. Am J Hum Biol 2004;16:125–34.
3. Wilder FV, Barrett JP, Farina EJ. Joint-specific prevalence of osteoarthritis of the hand. Osteoarthritis Cartilage 2006;14:953–7.
4. Brown RE, Zook EG, Russell RC, et al. Fingernail deformities secondary to ganglions of the distal interphalangeal joint (mucous cysts). Plast Reconstr Surg 1991;87:718–25.
5. Rangarathnam CS, Linscheid RL. Infected muous cyst of the finger. J Hand Surg Am 1984;9:245–7.
6. Epstein E. A simple technique for managing digital mucous cysts. Arch Dermatol 1979;115:1315–6.
7. Goldman JA, Goldman L, Jaffe MS, et al. Digital mucinous pseudocysts. Arthritis Rheum 1977;20:997–1002.
8. Rizzo M, Beckenbaugh RD. Treatment of mucous cysts of the fingers: review of 134 cases with minimum 2-year follow-up evaluation. J Hand Surg Am 2003;28:519–24.
9. Eaton RG, Dobranski AI, Littler JW. Marginal osteophyte excision in treatment of mucous cysts. J Bone Joint Surg Am 1973;55:570–4.
10. Lee HJ, Kim PT, Jeon IH, et al. Osteophyte excision without cyst excision for a mucous cyst of the finger. J Hand Surg Eur Vol 2014;39(3):258–61.
11. Kleinert HE, Kutz JE, Fishman JH, et al. Etiology and treatment of the so-called mucous cyst of the finger. J Bone Joint Surg Am 1972;54:1455–8.
12. Fritz GR, Stern PJ, Dickey M. Complications following mucous cyst excision. J Hand Surg Br 1977;22:222–5.
13. Kasdan ML, Stallings SP, Leis VM, et al. Outcome of surgical treated mucous cysts of the hand. J Hand Surg Am 1994;19:504–7.
14. Renfree KJ. Percutaneous in situ versus open arthrodesis of the distal interphalangeal joint. J Hand Surg Eur Vol 2015;40:379–83.
15. Dickson DR, Mehta SS, Nuttall D, et al. A systematic review of distal interphalangeal joint arthrodesis. J Hand Microsurg 2014;6:74–84.

16. Auzias P, Delarue R, Strouk G, et al. Distal interphalangeal joint arthrodesis with the intramedullary Lync® implant: prospective study of 22 cases. Hand Surg Rehabil 2019;38:114–20.

17. Melamed E, Polatsch DB, Beldner S, et al. Simulated distal interphalangeal joint fusion of the index and middle fingers in 0° and 20° of flexion: a comparison of grip strength and dexterity. J Hand Surg Am 2014;39:1986–91.

18. Schwartz DA, Peimer CA. Distal interphalangeal joint implant arthroplasty in a musician. J Hand Ther 1998;11:49–52.

19. Sierakowski A, Zweifel C, Sirotakova M, et al. Joint replacement in 131 painful osteoarthritis and post-traumatic distal interphalangeal joints. J Hand Surg Eur Vol 2012;37:304–9.

20. Wilgis EFS. Distal interphalangeal joint silicone interpositional arthroplasy of the hand. Clin Orthop Relat Res 1997;342:38–41.

21. Zimmerman NB, Suhey PV, Clark GL, et al. Silicone interpositional arthroplasty of the distal interphalangeal joint. J Hand Surg Am 1989;14: 882–7.

22. Zimmerman NB, Zimmerman SI, Wilgis EF. Distal interphalangeal joint silicone interpositional arthroplasy: surgical technique and functional outcome. Semin Arthroplasty 1991;2:153–7.

23. Brown LG. Distal interphalangeal joint flexible implant arthroplasty. J Hand Surg Am 1989;14: 653–6.

24. Snow JW, Boyes JG, Greider JL. Implant arthroplasty of the distal interphalangeal joint of the finger for osteoarthritis. Plast Reconstr Surg 1977; 60:558–60.

25. Rettig ME, Dassa G, Raskin KB. Volar plate arthroplasty of the distal interphalangeal joint. J Hand Surg Am 2001;26:940–4.

26. Aslam MZ, Ahmed SK, Fung B. New technique: tendon interposition arthroplasty in distal interphalangeal joint arthritis in Chinese population – new horizon for treatment. J Pak Med Assoc 2015; 65(11 Suppl 3):S8–11.

27. Lin EA, Papatheodorou LK, Sotereanos DG. Cheilectomy for treatment of symptomatic distal interphalangeal joint osteoarthritis: a review of 78 patients. J Hand Surg Am 2017;42(11):889–93.

Evaluation and Management of Scaphoid-Trapezium-Trapezoid Joint Arthritis

John C. Wu, MD*, James H. Calandruccio, MD

KEYWORDS

- Scaphoid-trapezium-trapezoid (STT) joint • Arthritis • Cause • Treatment • Outcomes
- Complications

KEY POINTS

- Degenerative arthritis at the articulation of the scaphoid, trapezium, and trapezoid (STT or triscaphe joint) is a relatively common degenerative disease of the wrist; isolated STT arthritis was found in 83% of cadaver wrists with an average age of 84 years.
- STT joint arthritis is not always symptomatic and often is an incidental finding on radiographs.
- The onset of symptoms, pain, loss of grip strength, and thumb function, usually is insidious and slowly progressive. Radial-sided wrist and thumb pain, swelling, and tenderness over the STT joint frequently are present.
- Suggested risk factors include age (>40 years of age), gender (more common and worse in women), heredity, and joint injury.
- Initial treatment is nonoperative; if nonoperative treatment fails, improvements in pain and motion can be obtained with a variety of operative procedures.

INTRODUCTION

Degenerative arthritis at the articulation of the scaphoid, trapezium, and trapezoid (STT or triscaphe joint) is a relatively common degenerative disease of the wrist and often is an incidental finding on radiographs. Isolated STT arthritis has been described in from 9% of 697 wrists in patients older than 50 years of age[1] to 83% in a cadaver study of 73 wrists with an average age of 84 years.[2] In an anatomic study of 393 cadaver wrists with an average age of 67 years, Viegas and colleagues[3] showed an average frequency of 20% of wrists with some degree of arthrosis at the STT articulation. Tomaino and colleagues[4] reported a scaphotrapeziotrapezoid arthritis rate of 62% by assessing the joint during trapeziectomy. By comparing the rate of arthritis seen during trapeziectomy to that assessed on preoperative radiographs, they concluded that radiographs were 44% sensitive and 86% specific for scaphotrapeziotrapezoid arthritis. Katzel and colleagues[5] found a 64% rate of scaphotrapeziotrapezoid arthritis in 896 radiographs.

The cause of STT arthritis is not completely understood, but multidirectional joint instability is thought to be a likely cause. The onset of symptoms, pain, loss of grip strength, and thumb function, usually is insidious and slowly progressive. Radial-sided wrist and thumb pain, swelling, and tenderness over the STT joint also may be present. Suggested risk factors include age (>40 years of age), gender (more common and worse in women), heredity, and joint injury.

Department of Orthopaedic Surgery and Biomedical Engineering, University of Tennessee-Campbell Clinic, 1211 Union Avenue, Suite 510, Memphis, TN 38104, USA
* Corresponding author.
E-mail address: john.cheeon.wu@gmail.com

Orthop Clin N Am 50 (2019) 497–508
https://doi.org/10.1016/j.ocl.2019.05.005

STT arthritis usually is not an isolated condition and frequently coexists with thumb trapeziometacarpal arthritis. Ferris and colleagues[1] noted an association between STT arthritis and static dorsal intercalated segment instability (DISI) deformity in their radiographic analysis of 697 wrists. More recently, Tay and colleagues[6] evaluated 24 wrists in 16 patients with STT arthritis and DISI deformity and noted that the scaphoid was extended in these patients rather than flexed as usually seen in DISI; they proposed that STT arthritis is a marker for nondissociative carpal instability.

ANATOMY

The scaphoid bridges the proximal and distal carpal rows on its radial side and articulates with the scaphoid fossa of the distal radius, the lunate, the capitate, the trapezium, and the trapezoid (Fig. 1). The scaphoid distal pole is dome shaped, which transfers load from the thumb and radial side of the hand to the radioscaphoid and scaphocapitate joints. Superior to and lateral to the scaphoid, the trapezium articulates with the scaphoid and the base of the first metacarpal through its unique saddle-shaped joint surface. Medially, the trapezoid articulates with the trapezium and the scaphoid as well as the capitate and also provides articulation for the base of the

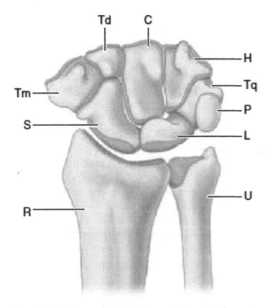

Fig. 1. Radiocarpal joint. C, capitate; H, hamate; L, lunate; P, pisiform; R, radius; S, scaphoid; Td, trapezoid; Tm, trapezium; Tq, triquetrum; U, ulna. (From Cannon DL. Wrist disorders. In: Azar FM, Beaty JH, Canale ST, editors. Campbell's operative orthopaedics, 13th edition. Philadelphia: Elsevier; 2017; with permission)

second metacarpal. Moritomo and colleagues[7] described the interfacet ridge of the distal scaphoid, which is aligned from radiodorsal to ulnar-volar and was present in 81% of cadaver wrists studied. The major ligaments of the STT articulation include the trapeziotrapezoid, the trapezoid-capitate, and the STT ligaments. The STT ligament has been identified as the major anatomic stabilizer of the STT joint. The capitate-trapezium ligament originates from the trapezium and inserts into the volar waist of the capitate and deepens the socket of the STT joint. The scaphotrapezial and trapeziotrapezoid volar ligaments help stabilize the joint, and the dorsolateral STT ligament stabilizes and links the joint to the rest of the midcarpus.

CLASSIFICATION

For many years, the radiographic classification designed by Crosby and colleagues[8] has been the most frequently used staging system: stage 0, normal joint; stage 1, slight joint space narrowing, and sclerosis; stage 2, marked joint space narrowing, osteophytes less than 2 mm; stage 3, osteophytes greater than 2 mm, subchondral cysts, and ankylosis. More recently, White and colleagues[9] described a classification system similar to that of Eaton and Littler[10] for carpometacarpal arthritis of the thumb (Fig. 2): stage 1, joint narrowing (compared with that of other intercarpal joints in the same radiograph), with or without subcortical sclerosis; stage 2, cystlike luciences with or without osteophytes; stage 3, complete joint space narrowing or bone-bone apposition without evident space within the cartilage.

CLINICAL PRESENTATION

Pain and weakness with grip strength reduction when performing tasks such as opening a jar are common complaints of patients with STT arthritis. Contrary to the dull ache often described with thumb carpometacarpal joint (CMC) joint arthritis, the pain often is sharp and occurs with certain particular movements.

Patients with isolated STT osteoarthritis may present with basilar thumb pain over the volarly located scaphoid tubercle or with dorsal radial-sided wrist pain. A painful bony prominence or fullness, corresponding to the STT joint, can be appreciated just distal to the radioscaphoid joint along the radial-dorsal side of the wrist and is similar in appearance to that seen in symptomatic scapholunate advanced collapse (SLAC) wrist deformity; however, the wrist dorsal prominence and synovitis associated with STT arthritis are

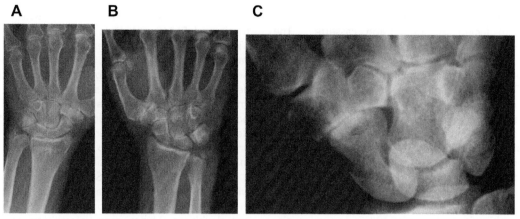

Fig. 2. Classification of STT arthritis. (A) Stage 1: narrowing of the joint space. (B) Stage 2: more severe narrowing, small osteophyte on the trapezium. (C) Stage 3: bone-bone apposition of the STT joint with subcortical sclerosis of the STT. In this case, the capitolunate joint space is abnormally narrow. (From White L, Clavijo J, Gilula LA, et al. Classification system for isolated arthritis of the scaphotrapeziotrapezoidal joint. Scand J Plast Reconstr Surg Hand Surg 2010;44(2):112–117; with permission.)

characteristically slightly more distal and ulnar than that associated with radioscaphoid degenerative processes. A radial grind test, in which the wrist is radially deviated to load the STT joint, also can elicit pain (Fig. 3).[11] Patients may present

with tendonitis along the flexor carpi radialis (FCR) tendon as it courses under the trapezial ridge to its distal insertion at the second metacarpal base. Degenerative changes, osteophyte formation, and local synovitis often can irritate this tendon, leading to tendonitis and possible rupture.

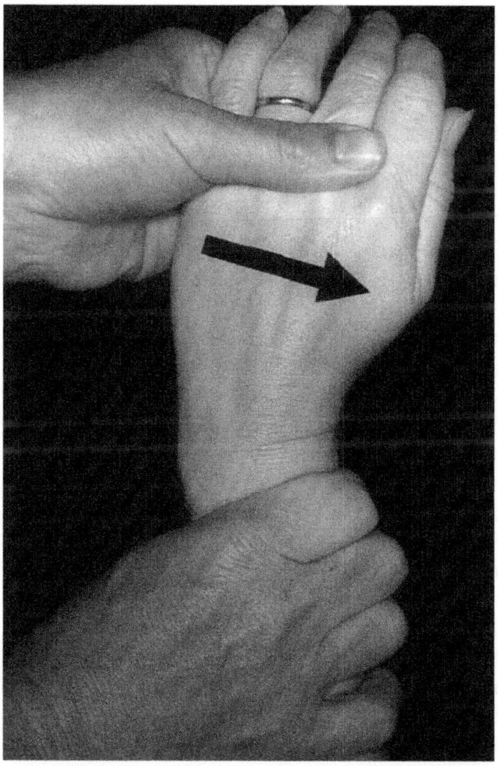

Differentiating between concomitant thumb CMC and STT arthritis can be difficult.[4] Concomitant trapeziometacarpal and STT osteoarthritis occurred in 60% of specimens in a cadaver study.[12] When both are present, the difficulty is determining if neither, one, or both joints are symptomatic and responsible for the patient's complaints. The basilar thumb pain in STT arthritis usually is more medial and proximal than the trapezial-metacarpal joint symptoms, which are commonly referred to the thenar eminence. In addition, isolated STT arthritic pain may not be exacerbated by the physical examination maneuvers often associated with thumb CMC arthritis, such as hyperadduction/hyperextension or the thumb CMC joint grind test.[4,13] These findings may help differentiate between STT joint pain and thumb CMC joint pain. Local injection of corticosteroid and lidocaine into either the thumb CMC joint or STT joint can be both diagnostic and therapeutic. Similar to thumb CMC osteoarthritis, not all patients with STT osteoarthritis are symptomatic,[14] and clinical examination may not correlate with the radiographic findings.

Fig. 3. Radial grind test. Pain is reproduced by passive radial deviation. Arrow indicates direction of force applied to hand. (From Davey PA, Belcher HJCR. Scapho-trapezio-trapezoidal joint osteoarthrosis. Curr Orthop 2001;15:220–228; with permission.)

RADIOGRAPHIC EVALUATION

Plain radiographs in 3 planes often are adequate for diagnosis of STT osteoarthritis.[14] A specific STT view can be obtained with the wrist in maximal extension and ulnar deviation with the palm facing the radiograph cassette.[15] The radiograph beam is directed perpendicular to and approximately 2.5 cm medial to the base of the thumb carpometacarpal joint (Fig. 4). The prevalence of STT osteoarthritis is relatively high as demonstrated in 1 study that evaluated radiographs in a cohort of patients presenting for any complaint.[16] Increasing age, presence of a scapho-lunate gap of more than 3 mm, and the presence of thumb CMC joint osteoarthritis were associated with STT osteoarthritis.

A wide range of data has been reported regarding the effectiveness of diagnosing STT arthritis with radiographs, but, in general, radiographs likely underestimate the true prevalence of STT arthritis. Brown and colleagues[12] found only a 39% agreement between radiographic and visual STT arthritis in cadaver specimens. Glickel and colleagues[17] found 66% concordance between intraoperative findings and plain radiographs.

CAUSE AND DIFFERENTIAL DIAGNOSIS OF SCAPHOID, TRAPEZIUM, AND TRAPEZOID ARTHRITIS

STT arthritis usually develops insidiously without apparent cause and often is associated with other several diagnoses. Ferris and colleagues[1] and Tay and colleagues[6] suggested an association between STT osteoarthritis and static DISI deformity. The causality of this relationship is unclear, and whether STT osteoarthritis leads to a DISI deformity or vice versa is speculative.

Chronic scapholunate (SL) ligament insufficiency leading to SLAC wrist and DISI deformity can result in STT arthritis,[16,18] despite reports of

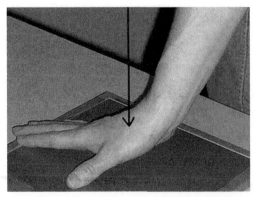

Fig. 4. STT radiographic view. (*From* Wollstein R, Wandzy N, Mastella DJ, et al. A radiographic view of the scaphotrapezium-trapezoid joint. J Hand Surg Am 2005;30(6):1162; with permission.)

an inverse relationship between STT osteoarthritis and SLAC wrist.[19] In this scenario, the STT ligaments (scapho-trapezium ligament and capitate-trapezium ligament, in particular) experience increased strain from the increased flexion moment seen on the scaphoid and proximal migration of the capitate through the SL gap.[18,20] Over time, this could result in STT joint degeneration and subsequent pain. Crystalline arthropathy also can lead to SLAC wrist deformity[21] and subsequent STT arthritis.[22]

Interestingly, isolated STT osteoarthritis, without SL widening, also can eventually result in a DISI deformity. DISI deformity often is associated with type I lunate morphology, where the lunate has a single articulation with the capitate.[23] STT arthritis may occur because type I lunate morphology is a less stable configuration for the proximal row,[24] whereas type II lunates have both a capitate and a hamate articulation and are more stable.[23] Shortening of the radial carpal column (scaphoid, trapezium, and trapezoid) secondary to cartilage thinning and bone loss at the STT joint may lead to scaphoid extension in an attempt to maintain carpal height. Eventually, the scaphoid is unable to maintain appropriate length from STT joint space loss, and the intermediate column (capitate and lunate) progressively collapses with resultant lunate extension and dorsal subluxation of the capitate.[25] With repetitive stress, the scaphoid-lunate ligament may attenuate to create a true DISI deformity.

Chronic midcarpal instability also can lead to STT arthritis, and the presence of midcarpal instability will impact surgical treatment; lateral radiographs should be carefully evaluated during the initial patient workup. A posterior drawer stress examination under fluoroscopy can be used to determine the presence of posterior midcarpal instability nondissociative, where the head of the capitate can subluxate or dislocate over the posterior lip of the lunate[26] (see Fig. 6). The dorsal midcarpal capsuloligamentous structures are hyperlax or insufficient, leading to dorsal instability. In theory, as the capitate subluxates dorsally, the scaphoid and lunate are forced into further extension, and shear stresses are increased at the STT joint. These increased and progressive repetitive loads exacerbate the STT joint degeneration.[26]

TREATMENT OF SCAPHOID, TRAPEZIUM, AND TRAPEZOID ARTHRITIS

Conservative treatment should be the initial treatment of STT arthritis and involves splinting, bracing, activity modification, anti-inflammatory medication, and steroid injections for pain relief. Failure of conservative treatment is the main indication for surgery. Treatment regimens should be tailored to the patient's physical demands, and surgical management plans may directly address the STT joint or concomitant instability patterns if present.

Distal Scaphoid Excision and Variations

Distal scaphoid excision with several variations has been described for idiopathic, symptomatic STT osteoarthritis as long as there is no midcarpal instability present. Advantages include a technically easier operation, less immobilization, faster recovery for the patient, and potentially less complications compared with arthrodesis.[26] The procedure does carry its own risks. Performing a distal scaphoid resection with midcarpal instability could further destabilize the carpus from "unlinking" the distal carpal row, resulting in a more pronounced DISI deformity.[26] Arthritic degeneration between the scaphoid, lunate, and capitate articulation is another contraindication because of load transfer from the STT joint to the central midcarpal joint after distal scaphoid excision.[27,28] A dorsal radial or palmar approach can be used,

with the palmar approach favored if FCR tendonitis is present to allow for examination of the tendon and possible tenolysis with excision of inflamed tenosynovium.[26] The plane of the scaphoid osteotomy is parallel to the trapezium-trapezoid proximal articular surface, with the wrist in neutral and the scaphoid at 45° to the radius. The original recommendation was for the excision to be no greater than one-quarter of the scaphoid (approximately 6 mm)[28]; however, more recent studies suggest that 3 mm of resection may be more appropriate.[29] Minimizing resection is important for preservation of the proximal origins of the dorsolateral STT and anteromedial scaphocapitate ligaments, which originate at both medial and lateral corners of the scaphoid tuberosity.

Several techniques have been described to fill the void after distal scaphoid excision and to maintain scaphoid stability and avoid excessive extension. FCR tendon interposition[30] and implant arthroplasty using a pyrocarbon implant[31–33] (Fig. 5) have been attempted. Tightening the volar radioscaphoid ligament, which functions as a tether, or tightening the dorsal scaphotrapezial capsule also helps avoid excessive scaphoid extension, although extension often occurs postoperatively to some degree.[26]

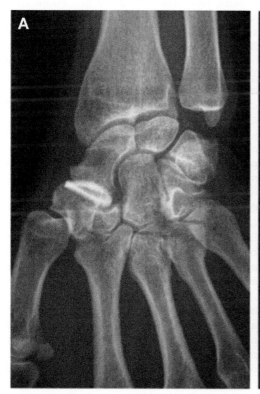
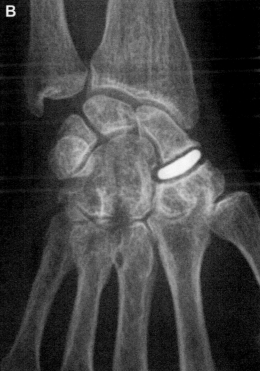

Fig. 5. Pyrocarbon implants for STT osteoarthritis. (*A*) Pyrocardan implant. (*B*) STPI implant. (*Reproduced from* Bellemère P. Pyrocarbon implants for the hand and wrist. Hand Surg Rehabil 2018;37(3):143. Copyright © 2018 published by Elsevier Masson SAS. All rights reserved.)

Arthroscopic techniques have been described for distal scaphoid excision.[34] Arthroscopic distal scaphoid excision may allow less immobilization and quicker recovery by minimizing local soft tissue dissection. A 1.9-mm arthroscope is recommended given the spatial constraints of the STT joint. The ulnar STT portal (ulnar to the tendons of the first dorsal compartment) is used as the working portal, and the midcarpal radial portal is used as the viewing portal (Fig. 6).[35] A volar portal can be used, as described by Carro and colleagues,[35] if there is difficulty visualizing the dorsoulnar portion of the STT joint. The sequence of the procedure is systematic and begins with a diagnostic arthroscopy, followed by joint debridement and synovectomy, and completed after resection of the distal scaphoid.[34] An open approach is still required if tendon interposition or implant arthroplasty is desired. A limited debridement of only synovitis, chondral flaps, and rim osteophytes, rather than distal scaphoid excision has also been described.[36]

Trapeziectomy and Variations

Total trapeziectomy is another option for treating STT osteoarthritic pain and is a popular procedure if there is symptomatic concomitant thumb CMC osteoarthritis. The ligament reconstruction, tendon interposition (LRTI), or some variant thereof, which is commonly used to treat thumb CMC osteoarthritic pain, also can be done for isolated recalcitrant STT arthritis.[37,38] Other variations include LRTI with partial

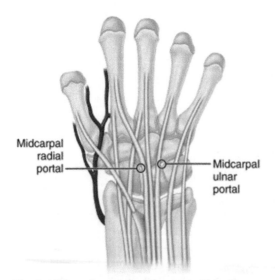

Fig. 6. Midcarpal portals for arthroscopy. (*From* Cannon DL. Wrist disorders. In: Azar FM, Beaty JH, Canale ST, editors. Campbell's operative orthopaedics, 13th edition. Philadelphia: Elsevier; 2017; with permission.)

excision of the proximal articular surface of the trapezoid (recommended 2 mm of resection) alone[39] or with interposition using a dermal graft[40] or the FCR tendon in the scaphotrapezoid space by placing a bone anchor into the trapezoid.[8,40] The rationale for treating STT pain with the trapezial resection techniques is to avoid scaphoid resection and minimize iatrogenic midcarpal instability[30]; however, carpal collapse and DISI deformity or abnormal extension of the scaphoid in the presence of a normal SL angle can still occur after trapeziectomy[41] (Fig. 7).

Scaphoid, Trapezium, and Trapezoid Arthrodesis

STT joint arthrodesis was initially described by Peterson and Lipscomb[42] in 1967 and was later popularized by Watson,[14,43,44] who advocated the procedure based on his successful results. Concerns over nonunion and ability to reproduce consistent results and outcomes have made some surgeons apprehensive of this technique. A contraindication is the presence of radioscaphoid joint degenerative changes, where fusion of the STT joints would lead to increased load transfer to this already arthritic joint. The key to the procedure is to fuse the bones in normal alignment, with the scaphoid angle occurring at 40° to 60° of flexion relative to the long axis of the radius, in the sagittal plane.[45] Restoring normal alignment optimizes postoperative range of motion by avoiding impingement that can occur if the scaphoid is extended. Watson and colleagues[42] recommended routine radial styloidectomy to avoid impingement. Construct options for fusion include Kirshner wire fixation, plates and screws, headless screws, and shape memory (compression) staples (Fig. 8).

OUTCOMES

Distal Scaphoid Excision

Excision is an effective surgical option that can provide reliable results and is a technically easier procedure, allows shorter immobilization, and avoids complications related to union.

In the study by Garcia-Elias and colleagues[46] of 21 wrists, 9 received no fibrous interposition and 12 wrists had capsular or tendon tissue to fill the defect. At follow-up, 13 wrists were pain free, whereas 8 had occasional mild discomfort. Grip was an average of 84%, and pinch strength was an average of 92% of the contralateral side. Mean range of movement was 118° of flexion-extension, with grip strength improved by 26% (P = .001) and pinch strength

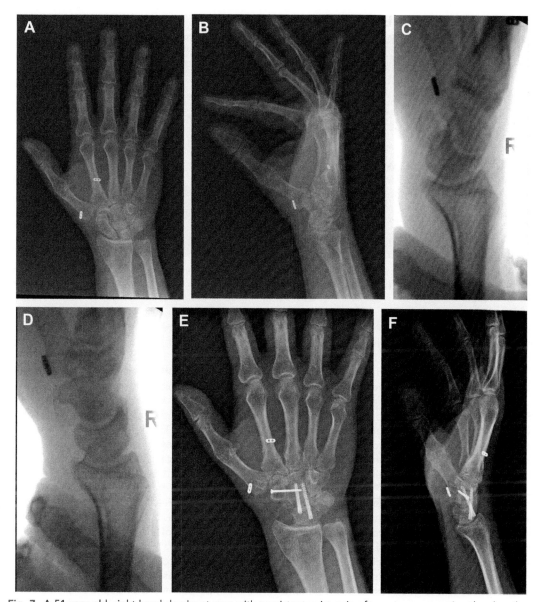

Fig. 7. A 51-year-old, right-hand-dominant man with persistent wrist pain after suture suspension thumb arthroplasty. (*A, B*) Residual scaphoid trapezoid joint space loss and dorsally subluxed capitate. (*C, D*) Intraoperative fluoroscopy shows easily reducible midcarpal joint. (*E, F*) After scaphoid excision and midcarpal fusion and supplementation of deficient trapezoid with scaphoid graft.

improved by 40% (*P* = .001). Of note, the wrists with no fibrous interposition showed significantly greater flexion-extension (mean 127°) than those with interposition (mean 113°) (*P* = .04).[27,46]

Wessels[47] reduced or eliminated pain in 54 of 56 patients with open excision of the distal 3 to 4 mm of the scaphoid and capsulorraphy.

Resection and Implant Arthroplasty
Most studies indicate that resection and implant arthroplasty have similar clinical results. Postoperative visual analogue scale (VAS) pain scores were 2.1 and 2.6 in the resection-only and implant groups, respectively. Pain scores decreased significantly in both groups (*P* = .007 and *P* = .01, respectively). The mean radiolunate (RL) angle increased from 14° to 30° in the resection-only group (*P* = .008). In the scaphoid trapezium pyrocarbon implant (STPI) group, there was an increase in the mean RL angle from 21° to 23°; however, this difference was not significant (*P* = .75).[32–34,48]

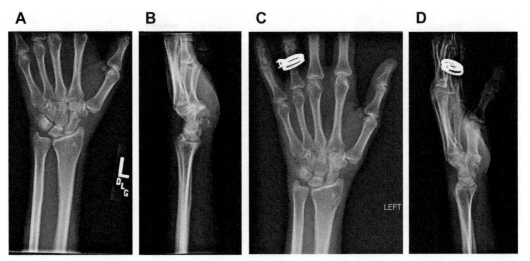

Fig. 8. A 53-year-old, right-hand-dominant woman with a ruptured FCR tendon and STT arthritis. (*A, B*) Appearance after allograft interposition of the scaphotrapezial joint. (*C, D*) After successful management of residudal pain with STT fusion.

Arthroscopic Treatment

In a study of 17 wrists, the average VAS score improved from 6.1 to 1.7 after surgery. The average grip strength improved from 18 to 19 kg. Pinch strength improved from 2.5 to 4.4 kg, and Patient-Related Wrist Evaluation (PRWE) score improved from 52 to 32.[29] Another study also demonstrated relief of pain in a series of 8 patients with isolated STT osteoarthritis, where 6 patients had complete relief and 1 patient had a decrease in symptoms.[49]

Ashwood and colleagues[36] reported good short-term follow-up (average follow-up 36 months) for pain relief in a series of 10 patients who underwent arthroscopic debridement of synovitis, chondral flaps and rim osteophytes, without distal scaphoid excision. VAS pain scores improved in all patients, with 9 patients reporting excellent to good results and 1 patient reporting fair results because of inability to achieve normal range of motion. The severity of arthritis was not noted in the study.

Ligament Reconstruction Tendon Interposition

Andrachuk and Yang[39] described their results of ligament reconstruction tendon interposition (LRTI) in 12 wrists for isolated STT joint osteoarthritis. Although their sample group was small and statistically insignificant, patients' symptoms, grip, and pinch strength were improved.

In 14 consecutive patients treated with trapeziectomy/LRTI for isolated scaphotrapeziotrapezoid osteoarthritis of the wrist, the median pain intensity was 0 on a 0 to 10 VAS, both at rest and with activity, mean grip strength averaged 24 kg, and pinch strength averaged 5 kg.[38] The disabilities of the arm, shoulder, and hand (DASH) score was 16, and a modified Mayo Wrist Score was 84. Correlation between the degree of scaphotrapezoid osteoarthritis and pain at rest, pain with activity, and DASH score was not significant. These findings suggest that trapeziectomy/LRTI is an effective procedure for treating isolated scaphotrapeziotrapezoid osteoarthritis. In comparison to Andrachuk and Yang's results,[39] these results suggest that the addition of partial trapezoid excision is not imperative for effective treatment of isolated STT osteoarthritis. Trapeziectomy and LRTI have been reported not to affect carpal alignment.[38]

Tomaino and colleagues[4] studied 37 patients with trapezial excision and compared the results between 23 patients with trapezial excision and proximal trapezoid excision for combined CMC and STT joint osteoarthritis with those of 14 patients with trapeziectomy only for isolated CMC joint osteoarthritis. There was no increased morbidity with the combined procedure. The differences in postoperative grip and pinch strengths between the 2 groups were not statistically significant. Trapeziectomy and partial trapezoidal excision produced good pain relief and motion with low morbidity and complication rates.

Scaphoid, Trapezium, and Trapezoid Arthrodesis

In Watson and Hempton's series,[43] triscaphe fusion was performed using three 0.045-inch Kirschner wires in 13 patients, 7 of whom had degenerative changes of the STT joint.

Outcomes were good overall, with a flexion-extension arc of 104° and stated pain relief. Watson and Hempton[43] produced one of the earliest comprehensive reports on the operative treatment of STT arthritis in 1980. This arthrodesis was reported to "leave the wrist strong with minimal loss of motion." Another description of 5 STT arthrodeses for degenerative joint disease, with an average of 3 years of follow-up, reported fair patient satisfaction.[8]

Meier and colleagues[50] treated 111 patients with STT fusion, 83 of whom were available for evaluation at an average follow-up of 4 years. Eight patients of the STT osteoarthritis group (n = 11) had the best Mayo Wrist Score (71 points) compared with the other groups. In these patients, grip strength averaged 84% of the opposite hand and wrist flexion-extension averaged 90% compared with the preoperative motion. Pain at rest and activity decreased to 78% and 63%, respectively. Other studies have shown STT joint arthrodesis to be a valid therapeutic treatment with satisfactory results.[51]

STT arthrodesis is associated with several complications that likely limit its universal use for treatment of recalcitrant STT osteoarthritic pain. The overall complication rate in a large series of patients (800 wrists) with STT fusion was 13.4%.[38]

COMPLICATIONS OF OPERATIVE TREATMENT

In general, the surgical approach can place surrounding sensory nerves and the radial artery at risk.[47] One study noted superficial radial neuromas in situ in 7 patients out of 800, who presumably required surgical treatment.[52]

Flexor Tendon Rupture
Flexor tendon rupture has been reported after distal scaphoid excision. Deren and colleagues[53] suggested that a sharp bony remnant of the distal scaphoid eroded through the volar capsule, which led to attritional rupture of the adjacent flexor digitorum profundus and flexor digitorum superficialis tendons to the index finger. They recommended smoothing any sharp bony prominence after the osteotomy to avoid this complication. FPL rupture can also occur through this same mechanism.[27]

Dorsal Intercalated Segment Instability and Midcarpal Misalignment
A DISI deformity can occur after distal scaphoid excision, especially if midcarpal instability is present. Garcia-Elias and colleagues[28] found that distal scaphoid excision consistently led DISI deformity in their series but did not find any correlation between the patients' functional outcomes and the DISI deformity. Iida and colleagues[29] found an increased carpal deformity (defined as a capitate-lunate angle >15°) when greater than 3 mm of distal scaphoid was excised. There has been a slightly lower reported incidence of carpal misalignment with the use of a pyrocarbon implant.[32,48] In theory, by filling the resected space, the implant can possibly restore the flexion moment of the scaphoid to neutralize the lunate from the extension forces exerted by the triquetrum. Pequignot and colleagues[48] found that angular measurements were not altered in patients treated with a scaphoid-trapezial pyrocarbon implant; however, implants may be associated with higher rates of complications with an 8% to 10% rate of implant dislocation.[48] Alternatively, trapeziectomy with LRTI did not affect carpal alignment in a series published by Langenhan and colleagues.[38]

Nonunion
Nonunion was the most common complication (4%) in a series of 36 patients published by Watson and colleagues.[44] A subsequent larger series also published by Watson and colleagues[52] reported a relatively low nonunion rate; however, this has not been reproduced by others. Another group found a much higher nonunion rate with 5 out of 19 wrists (26%) treated with STT arthrodesis. Four of these wrists required revision surgery.[54] Subsequent studies reported nonunion rates of 24%[55] and 16%.[56] Vascularized bone graft from the radius has been used to try to minimize the probability of nonunion, with reported radiologic union reliably occurring at 8 to 12 weeks postoperatively.[57]

Radial Styloid Impingement
Symptomatic radial styloid impingement can occur after STT arthrodesis secondary to altered carpal kinematics and inability of the scaphoid to flex and clear with radial deviation. One study reported radial impingement in 31 out of 93 STT fusions (33%), with a higher incidence seen in patients who were treated for rotatory subluxation of the scaphoid.[58] Partial radial styloidectomy provided resolution of pain and impingement, leading the investigators to recommend this to be performed routinely with all STT arthrodesis.[27,52,58]

Adjacent Joint Arthrosis and Degeneration
Adjacent joint arthrosis and degeneration are concerns after any arthrodesis. Fortin and

Louis[56] found that progressive arthrosis of the radial-carpal and trapezial-metacarpal joint occurred in a study of 14 patients with an average follow-up of 5 years after STT fusion. There was arthrosis in 6 patients at the radiocarpal joint and 4 patients at the trapezial-metacarpal joint. Three of these 10 patients underwent additional surgery, including carpometacarpal arthroplasty and radiocarpal fusion. The investigators noted that fusion of the scaphoid within acceptable alignment did not preclude development of arthrosis.

Reflex Sympathetic Dystrophy

Reflex sympathetic dystrophy can occur after STT arthrodesis and was reported in 29 patients (3.6%) in his series of 800 patients. These patients were treated with conservative management, and long-term outcome of this complication was not provided.[52]

SUMMARY

Degenerative arthritis at the articulation of the STT (or triscaphe joint) is a relatively common degenerative disease of the wrist. Pain and weakness with grip strength and when performing tasks such as opening a jar are common complaints of patients with STT arthritis. Conservative treatment should be the initial treatment of STT arthritis and involves splinting, bracing, activity modification, anti-inflammatory medication, and steroid injections for pain relief. Failure of conservative treatment is the main indication for surgery, which may include distal scaphoid excision, with or without filling of the void after excision, trapeziectomy, STT arthrodesis, or STT implant arthroplasty. Improvements in pain and motion can be obtained with most of these described techniques, although none is without a set of subsequent complications, which may be difficult to salvage with a secondary operation. Hence, initial conservative approaches to patients with STT arthritis are advised, and the anticipated surgical outcomes, including technique-specific complications, are discussed with appropriate surgical candidates.

REFERENCES

1. Ferris BD, Dunnett W, Lavelle JR. An association between scaphotrapezio-trapezoid osteoarthritis and static dorsal intercalated segment instability. J Hand Surg Br 1994;19(3):338–9.
2. Bhatia A, Pisoh T, Touam C, et al. Incidence and distribution of scaphotrapezo-trapezoidal arthritis in 73 fresh cadaveric wrists. Ann Chir Main Memb Super 1996;15(4):220–5.
3. Viegas SF, Patterson RM, Hokanson JA, et al. Wrist anatomy: incidence, distribution, and correlation of anatomic variations, tears, and arthrosis. J Hand Surg Am 1993;18:463–75.
4. Tomaino MM, Vogt M, Weiser R. Scaphotrapezoid arthritis: prevalence in thumbs undergoing trapezium excision arthroplasty and efficacy of proximal trapezoid excision. J Hand Surg Am 1999;24:1220–4.
5. Katzel EB, Bielicka D, Shakir S, et al. Carpal and scaphotrapeziotrapezoid arthritis in patients with carpometacarpal arthritis. Plast Reconstr Surg 2016;137:1793–8.
6. Tay SC, Moran SL, Shin AY, et al. The clinical implications of scaphotrapezium-trapezoidal arthritis with associated carpal instability. J Hand Surg Am 2007;32(1):47–54.
7. Moritomo H, Viegas SF, Nakamura K, et al. The scaphotrapezio-trapezoidal joint. Part 1: an anatomic and radiographic study. J Hand Surg 2000;25A:899–910.
8. Crosby EB, Linscheid RL, Dobyns JH. Scaphotrapezial trapezoidal arthrosis. J Hand Surg Am 1978;3:223–34.
9. White L, Clavijo J, Gilula LA, et al. Classification system for isolated arthritis of the scaphotrapeziotrapezoidal joint. Scand J Plast Reconstr Surg Hand Surg 2010;44:112–7.
10. Eaton EG, Littler JW. Ligament reconstruction for the painful thumb carpometacarpal joint. J Bone Joint Surg Am 1975;55:1655–66.
11. Davey PA, Belcher HJCR. Scapho-trapezio-trapezoidal joint osteoarthrosis. Curr Orthop 2001;15: 220–8.
12. Brown GD III, Roh MS, Strauch RJ, et al. Radiography and visual pathology of the osteoarthritic scaphotrapezio-trapezoidal joint, and its relationship to trapeziometacarpal osteoarthritis. J Hand Surg Am 2003;28(5):739–43.
13. Wolf JM. Treatment of scaphotrapezio-trapezoid arthritis. Hand Clin 2008;24:301–6.
14. Wollstein R, Watson HK. Scaphotrapeziotrapezoid arthrodesis for arthritis. Hand Clin 2005;21:539–43.
15. Wollstein R, Wandzy N, Mastella DJ, et al. A radiographic view of the scaphotrapezium-trapezoid joint. J Hand Surg Am 2005;30:1161–3.
16. Scordino LE, Bernstein J, Nakashian M, et al. Radiographic prevalence of scaphotrapeziotrapezoid osteoarthritis. J Hand Surg Am 2014;39:1677–82.
17. Glickel SZ, Kornstein AN, Eaton RG. Long-term follow-up of trapeziometacarpal arthroplasty with coexisting scaphotrapezial disease. J Hand Surg Am 1992;17:612–20.
18. Roberts C, Porter M, Wines AP, et al. The association of scapho-trapezio-trapezoid osteoarthritis and scapholunate dissociation. Hand Surg 2006; 11:135–41.

19. Wollstein R, Clavijo J, Gilula LA. Osteoarthritis of the wrist STT joint and radiocarpal joint. Arthritis 2012;2012:242159.

20. van der Westhuizen J, Mennen U. A working classification for the management of scapho-trapezium-trapeziodosteo-arthritis. Hand Surg 2010;15:203–10.

21. Doherty W, Lovallo JL. Scapholunate advanced collapse pattern of arthritis in calcium pyrophosphate deposition disease of the wrist. J Hand Surg Am 1993;18:1095–8.

22. Saffar P. Chondrocalcinosis of the wrist. J Hand Surg Br 2004;29:486–93.

23. McLean JM, Turner PC, Bain GI, et al. An association between lunate morphology and scaphoid-trapezium-trapezoid arthritis. J Hand Surg Eur Vol 2009;34:778–82.

24. Galley I, Bain GI, McLean JM. Influence of lunate type on scaphoid kinematics. J Hand Surg Am 2007;32:842–7.

25. Lluch AL, Garcia-Elias M, Lluch AB. Arthroplasty of the scaphoid-trapezium-trapezoid and carpometacarpal joints. Hand Clin 2013;29:57.

26. Garcia-Elias M. Excisional arthroplasty for scaphotrapeziotrapezoidal osteoarthritis. J Hand Surg Am 2011;36:516–20.

27. Deans VM, Naqui Z, Muir LT. Scaphotrapeziotrapezoidal joint osteoarthritis: a systematic review of surgical treatment. J Hand Surg Asian Pac Vol 2017;22:1–9.

28. Garcia-Elias M, Lluch A, Saffar P. Distal scaphoid excision in scaphoid-trapezium-trapezoid arthritis. Tech Hand Up Extrem Surg 1999;3:169–73.

29. Iida A, Omokawa S, Kawamura K, et al. Arthroscopic distal scaphoid resection for isolated scaphotrapeziotrapezoid osteoarthritis. J Hand Surg Am 2019;44:337.e1-7.

30. Moreno R, Bhandari L. FCT interposition arthroplasty for concomitant STT and CMC arthritis. Tech Hand Up Extrem Surg 2019;23:10–3.

31. Gauthier E, Truffandier MV, Gaisne E, et al. Treatment of scaphotrapezio-trapezoid osteoarthritis with the Pyrocardan® implant: results with a minimum follow-up of 2 years. Hand Surg Rehabil 2017;36:113–21.

32. Marcuzzi A, Ozben H, Russomando A. Treatment of scaphotrapezial trapezoidal osteoarthritis with resection of the distal pole of the scaphoid. Acta Orthop Traumatol Turc 2014;48:431–6.

33. Low AK, Edmunds IA. Isolated scapotraeziotrapezoid osteoarthritis: preliminary results of treatment using a pyrocarbon implant. Hand Surg 2007;12:73–7.

34. Pegoli L, Pozzi A. Arthroscopic management of scaphoid-trapezium-trapezoid joint arthritis. Hand Clin 2017;33:813–7.

35. Carro LP, Golano P, Farinas O, et al. The radial portal for scaphotrapezio-trapezoid arthroscopy. Arthroscopy 2003;19:547–53.

36. Ashwood N, Bain GI, Fogg O. Results of arthroscopic debridement for isolated scaphotrapeziotrapezoid arthritis. J Hand Surg Am 2003;28:729.

37. Wolf JM, Delaronde S. Current trends in nonoperative and operative treatment of trapeziometacarpal osteoarthritis: a survey of US hand surgeons. J Hand Surg Am 2012;37:77–82.

38. Langenhan R, Hohendorff B, Probst A. Trapeziectomy and ligament reconstruction tendon interposition for isolated scaphotrapeziotrapezoid osteoarthritis of the wrist. J Hand Surg Eur Vol 2014;39:833–7.

39. Andrachuk J, Yang SS. Modified total trapezial and partial trapezoidal excision and ligament reconstruction tendon interposition reduces symptoms in isolated scaphotrapezial-trapezoid arthritis of the wrist. J Hand Surg Eur Vol 2012;37:637–41.

40. Warganich T, Shin AY. A technique for the management of concomitant scaphotrapezoid arthritis in patients with thumb metacarpotrapezial arthritis: interposition arthroplasty with a capitate suture anchor. Tech Hand Up Extrem Surg 2017;21:71–4.

41. Yuan BJ, Moran SL, Tay SC, et al. Trapeziectomy and carpal collapse. J Hand Surg Am 2009;34:219.

42. Peterson HA, Lipscomb PR. Intercarpal arthrodesis. Arch Surg 1967;95:127–34.

43. Watson HK, Hempton RF. Limited wrist arthrodesis. I. The triscaphoid joint. J Hand Surg Am 1980;5:320–7.

44. Minamikawa Y, Peimer CA, Yamaguchi T, et al. Ideal scaphoid angle for intercarpal arthrodesis. J Hand Surg Am 1992;17:370–5.

45. Watson HK, Weinzsweig J, Guidera PM, et al. One thousand intercarpal arthrodesis. J Hand Surg Br 1999;24:307–15.

46. Garcia-Elias M, Lluch AL, Farreres A, et al. Resection of the distal scaphoid for scaphotrapeziotrapezoid osteoarthritis. J Hand Surg Br 1999;24:448–52.

47. Wessels KD. Arthroplasty of osteoarthritic triscaphe (distal scaphoid) joint. Oper Orthop Traumatol 2004;16:48–58.

48. Pequignot JP, D'asnieres de Veigy L, Allieu Y. Arthroplasty for scaphotrapezio-trapezoidal arthrosis using a pyrolytic carbon implant. Preliminary results. Chir Main 2005;24:148–52 [in French].

49. Normand J, Desmoineaux P, Boisrenoult P, et al. The arthroscopic distal pole resection of the scaphoid: clinical results in STT arthritis. Chir Main 2012;31:13.

50. Meier R, Prommersberger KJ, Krimmer H. Scaphotrapezio-trapezoid arthrodesis (triscaphe arthrodesis). Handchir Mikrochir Plast Chir 2003;35:323–7.

51. Srinivasan VB, Matthews JP. Results of scaphotrapeziotrapezoid fusion for isolated idiopathic arthritis. J Hand Surg Br 1996;21:378–80.

52. Watson HK, Wollstein R, Joseph E, et al. Scaphotrapeziotrapezoid arthrodesis: a follow-up study. J Hand Surg Am 2003;28:397.

53. Deren ME, Mitchell CH, Weiss AC. Flexor tendon ruptures after distal scaphoid excision for scapho-trapeziotrapezoid osteoarthritis. Hand (N Y) 2017; 12:NP152–6.

54. Frykman EB, Ekenstam FA, Wadin K. Triscaphoid arthrodesis and its complications. J Hand Surg Am 1988;13:844–9.

55. McAuliffe JA, Dell PC, Jaffe R. Complications of intercarpal arthrodesis. J Hand Surg Am 1993;18: 1121–8.

56. Fortin PT, Louis DS. Long-term follow-up of scaphoid-trapezium-trapezoid arthrodesis. J Hand Surg Am 1993;18:675–81.

57. Nemoto T, Inagaki K. Scaphotrapeziotrapezoid fusion for arthritis with vascularized bone grafting from the radius. J Hand Surg Eur Vol 2011;36: 820–1.

58. Rogers WD, Watson HK. Radial styloid impinge-ment after triscaphe arthrodesis. J Hand Surg Am 1989;14(2 Pt 1):297–301.

Shoulder and Elbow

Management of the B2 Glenoid in Glenohumeral Osteoarthritis

Siddhant K. Mehta, MD, PhD, Alexander W. Aleem, MD*

KEYWORDS

- Walch B2 glenoid • Biconcave glenoid • Eccentric corrective reaming • Bone grafting
- Augmented glenoid • Reverse shoulder arthroplasty

KEY POINTS

- The B2 glenoid is characterized by an eccentric wear pattern and is associated with posterior bone loss, increased glenoid retroversion, a biconcave appearance, and posterior humeral head subluxation.
- Surgical reconstruction of the B2 shoulder with anatomic total shoulder arthroplasty is challenging but can be achieved through several techniques, including eccentric corrective glenoid reaming, bone grafting, and augmented glenoid implants.
- In cases of extreme glenoid retroversion, bone loss, and humeral head subluxation, reverse shoulder arthroplasty, even in cuff-intact shoulders, is a surgical option to alleviate pain and restore function.

INTRODUCTION

Degenerative arthritis of the shoulder results in a significant burden to the patient with respect to pain, level of function, and quality of life. As the disorder associated with glenohumeral osteoarthritis has become better understood and defined, certain features of glenoid morphology, namely an asymmetric glenoid wear pattern with glenoid bone loss, excessive glenoid retroversion, and posterior humeral head subluxation, have been identified to be particularly challenging at the time of surgical reconstruction. These characteristics that are associated with the B2 glenoid can be surgically managed in several ways, including arthroscopic debridement, hemiarthroplasty, anatomic total shoulder arthroplasty (TSA) with eccentric reaming, bone grafting, augmented glenoid implants, and reverse TSA (RTSA). This review article describes each of these techniques and presents the current available literature in an effort to guide evidence-based decisions in the management of the B2 glenoid deformity.

Glenoid Morphology

Neer[1,2] first described a spectrum of glenohumeral changes in primary osteoarthritis and noted that advanced cases had a posteriorly sloped glenoid and associated posterior subluxation of the humeral head. A formal classification of glenoid morphology was later developed by Walch and colleagues[3,4] based on preoperative computed tomography (CT) scans (**Fig. 1**). The type A glenoid shows a well-centered humeral head and concentric central erosion. In contradistinction, the type B glenoid is characterized by posterior humeral head subluxation with asymmetric loading. The B1 subgroup has posterior joint space narrowing, subchondral sclerosis, and osteophytes without erosion, whereas the B2 subgroup is characterized by a posterior wear pattern, giving a biconcave glenoid appearance. The erosion pattern typically

---

Disclosure: The authors have nothing to disclose.

Shoulder and Elbow Surgery, Department of Orthopaedic Surgery, Washington University School of Medicine, 660 South Euclid Avenue, Campus Box 8233, Saint Louis, MO 63110, USA

* Corresponding author.

E-mail address: aleema@wustl.edu

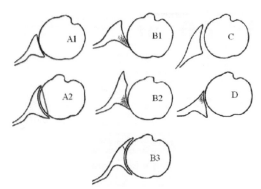

Fig. 1. The modified Walch classification of the glenoid in primary glenohumeral osteoarthritis. (*From* Bercik MJ, Kruse K, II, Yalizis M, et al. A modification to the Walch classification of the glenoid in primary glenohumeral osteoarthritis using three-dimensional imaging. J Shoulder Elbow Surg 2016;25(10):1602; with permission.)

present in the B2 glenoid involves the posteroinferior quadrant with a biconcavity demarcation line from posterosuperior to anteroinferior.[5–7] The type C glenoid is defined by retroversion measuring more than 25°, not caused by erosion that is dysplastic in origin.[3,4] In this group, the humeral head is typically well centered or only slightly posteriorly subluxated. The B3 glenoid was described by Bercik and colleagues[4] based on three-dimensional (3D) CT reconstructions as a monocave, posteriorly worn glenoid with at least 15° of retroversion or at least 70% posterior humeral head subluxation, or both. Furthermore, the type D glenoid is characterized by anterior humeral head subluxation or glenoid anteversion.[4] Most recently, a B0 subgroup was added to the classification to describe a preosteoarthritic posterior humeral head subluxation.[8]

Quantifying the B2 Glenoid

Certain objective measures allow quantification of the B2 glenoid deformity, namely glenoid version and humeral head subluxation. Glenoid version can be measured on axial CT images, as previously described by Friedman and colleagues.[9] A reference line for the transverse scapular axis (Friedman line) is drawn from the tip of the medial border of the scapula to the center of the glenoid fossa. A line perpendicular to the Friedman line represents neutral glenoid version. The angle formed by this neutral line and a line connecting the anterior and posterior margins of the glenoid represents the degrees of version. If the posterior margin of the glenoid is medial to this neutral line, then the definition of glenoid retroversion is met and the measured

version angle is recorded as a negative number. Specific to the B2 glenoid is the biconcavity, which can make quantifying the degree of retroversion challenging. Rouleau and colleagues[10] studied several measurement strategies and described 3 additional reference lines to better assess version of the B2 glenoid. The paleoglenoid is the original glenoid, the neoglenoid is the posterior erosion surface, and the intermediate glenoid is a line connecting the anterior and posterior margins. Measuring humeral head subluxation is also useful in quantifying the B2 glenoid, because it has been suggested as the eventual cause of posterior glenoid erosion.[6,11] This measurement is commonly performed by measuring the percentage of the humeral head that lies posterior to the Friedman line on axial CT cuts, representing the humeral scapular alignment. This method has been shown to be particularly useful in the setting of a B2 glenoid.[12] Posterior humeral head subluxation has been shown to be associated with poorer outcomes after shoulder arthroplasty.

TREATMENT OPTIONS

The goals of surgical management of the B2 glenoid include alleviation of shoulder pain and restoration of upper extremity function. This outcome can be accomplished in several ways, including arthroscopic debridement as well as TSA, using a variety of techniques. When performing surgical reconstruction, the primary goal is to restore the functional anatomy of the glenohumeral joint and to optimize long-term durability of the prosthetic implants. The challenges faced when reconstructing the B2 glenoid are compromised glenoid bone stock, excessive glenoid retroversion, and posterior humeral head subluxation. If not appropriately addressed, these can lead to component malpositioning, perforation or fracture at the time of glenoid implantation, or postoperative instability, all of which can affect implant longevity and clinical outcome.

Given that no single treatment option has been proved to be superior, each technique should be carefully considered based on several factors, including patient characteristics, level of activity, bone quality, and degree of deformity. The potential risks and theoretic benefits should be weighed, and postoperative expectations should be discussed in great detail before proceeding with any single management strategy. The advantages and disadvantages of the various surgical management strategies for the B2 glenoid are summarized in Table 1.

Table 1
Surgical management of the B2 glenoid

Technique	Advantages	Disadvantages
Arthroscopic debridement	Minimally invasive	Not definitive
	Temporarily delays need for arthroplasty	Unpredictable duration of symptomatic relief
Hemiarthroplasty	Avoidance of glenoid implant–related complications	Inferior pain relief and functional outcomes
TSA + eccentric reaming	Allows for version correction up to approximately 15°	Loss of glenoid bone stock with reaming
		Potential for glenoid vault perforation/glenoid fracture
TSA + bone grafting	Allows for version correction	Technically challenging
	Enhances glenoid bone stock	Graft-related complications
TSA + augmented glenoid	Limited reaming (medialization) required	Requires removal of posteriorly located high-quality bone
	Preservation of bone stock	Implant-associated costs
RSA	Correction of instability afforded by a constrained design	Unpredictable longevity in younger patients
		Limited revision options

Arthroscopic Debridement

Arthroscopic joint debridement with or without a capsular release has been used as a minimally invasive method to achieve pain relief and improve function in select patients who are considered poor arthroplasty candidates because of young age or high activity level. It is offered as an alternative to arthroplasty to patients who present with pain, stiffness, or mechanical symptoms, to serve as a temporary solution until a time when arthroplasty is more suitable.

Although several investigators have reported acceptable outcomes after arthroscopic debridement for advanced glenohumeral arthritis, including reduced pain, improved function, and a delay in the need for shoulder arthroplasty, the duration of relief is brief and failure rates may be as high as 30%.[13,14] Spiegl and colleagues[15] performed a Markov decision analysis, a level II economic and decision analysis, and reported that arthroscopic management was the preferred treatment strategy for patients less than 47 years of age, whereas TSA was preferred in patients more than 66 years of age. This finding was corroborated by Mitchell and colleagues,[16,17] who identified that age greater than 50 years was a risk factor for failure of arthroscopic management, defined as progression to total joint arthroplasty.

The goal of arthroscopic debridement is to remove any loose bodies, remove frayed tissues,

resect synovitis, and recontour loose soft tissues to a stable margin, such that there is a reduction in mechanical symptoms and pain.[13,18,19] In addition, a capsular release allows improved range of motion and function.[14,19] If significant biceps disorder is noted, a biceps tenotomy or tenodesis can also be considered to improve postoperative pain relief.[13,20,21] Millet and colleagues[22–24] recently described the comprehensive arthroscopic management (CAM) procedure to address glenohumeral osteoarthritis. The CAM procedure includes the procedures mentioned earlier but also includes humeral osteoplasty and axillary nerve neurolysis to remove the inferior humeral osteophyte and decompress the axillary nerve, as well as microfracture for high-grade chondral lesions.

Survivorship and patient-reported outcomes after CAM procedures with a minimum follow-up of 5 years have been published by Mitchell and colleagues.[16] They analyzed 47 shoulders in 44 consecutive patients who underwent the procedure, with a mean age of 52 years (range, 27–68 years). All patients were noted to be recreational athletes. Twelve of 47 shoulders (26%) progressed to arthroplasty at a mean of 2.6 years. Survivorship was observed as 95.6% at 1 year, 86.7% at 3 years, and 76.9% at 5 years. Walch type B2 or C glenoid morphology and preoperative joint space narrowing of less than 2 mm on anteroposterior or Grashey view were noted to be a significant risk factors for failure and progression to arthroplasty. Notably, 2 patients required a secondary arthroscopic surgery (capsular release for stiffness at 5.6 months; revision CAM procedure at 7.9 years) and were not considered failures. Most recently, Mitchell and colleagues[17] investigated the preoperative factors predictive of treatment failure after the CAM procedure. They reviewed 107 shoulders in 99 patients with a mean age of 52 years (range, 29–77 years). Seventeen of 107 shoulders (15.8%) progressed to arthroplasty. Among the preoperative factors that were associated with progression to arthroplasty after the CAM procedure were age older than 50 years, radiographically more severe arthritis as measured by the Kellgren-Lawrence grade, narrower joint space, and Walch type B2 or C glenoid anatomy. Importantly, the relative risk of progression to arthroplasty was approximately 6 times higher in patients with a type B2 or type C glenoid morphology compared with A1, A2, or B1 types.

Although arthroscopic management for glenohumeral arthritis may be a reasonable alternative to arthroplasty in select patients, those with a type B2 glenoid have a significantly higher risk of progression to arthroplasty. As such, expectations regarding improvement and duration of pain relief and functional outcomes are critical, and the ultimate decision regarding surgical management should be shared between the surgeon and patient.

Hemiarthroplasty

Hemiarthroplasty for glenohumeral arthritis is typically performed in young, high-demand, active patients in whom there is concern regarding the longevity of glenoid implantation. Hemiarthroplasty can also be considered in patients with poor glenoid bone stock that would preclude appropriate glenoid component stability. Although outcome studies of hemiarthroplasty performed specifically for type B2 glenoids are not available in the current literature, there are several studies that provide further insight regarding its limited role in the management of such patients.

Levine and colleagues[25] performed a retrospective review of 31 shoulders in 30 patients after hemiarthroplasty for glenohumeral arthritis. They showed inferior functional outcomes of hemiarthroplasty in shoulders with primary osteoarthritis that showed characteristic posterior bone loss and humeral head subluxation, with satisfactory results achieved in only 63% of cases. In contrast, a satisfactory outcome was achieved in 86% of cases with a concentric erosion pattern. In a longer-term follow-up study, Levine and colleagues[26] reported 13% satisfactory results in eccentric glenoids compared with 42% in concentric glenoids.

The ream-and-run technique has been popularized by Matsen and colleagues.[27] In this procedure, after the glenoid is reamed to create a concentric socket, a hemiarthroplasty is performed. Lynch and colleagues[28] reported self-assessed pain and functional outcomes in patients who underwent the ream-and-run procedure with a mean follow-up of 2.7 years. Of the 34 shoulders, 4 (12%) went on to develop progressive posterior erosion and 6 (18%) had recurrent posterior erosion. Similarly, Gilmer and colleagues[29] assessed the prognostic factors that are associated with improved function and comfort after the ream-and-run procedure in 162 patients with a minimum follow-up of 2 years. They found that 124 patients (76%) were improved by a minimal clinically important difference, 16 patients (10%) were not improved, 22 patients (14%) required a repeat surgery of which 7 were revised to TSA. No patients were observed to have posterior instability. However, among the biconcave glenoids, 23% had minimal clinically important difference improvement in functional scores, 38% were not improved, and 14% required revision. Weldon and colleagues[30] showed that, biomechanically, resection of the labral tissues and glenoid cartilage result in decreased stability, and concentric glenoid reaming helps restore glenohumeral stability. In light of these studies, hemiarthroplasty with or without glenoid reaming in patients with B2 glenoid morphology should be performed with caution.

Anatomic Total Shoulder Arthroplasty

Surgical reconstruction of the B2 shoulder with anatomic TSA is challenging but can be achieved through several techniques that aid in glenoid version correction and recentering the posteriorly subluxated humeral head. These advanced surgical techniques include eccentric corrective glenoid reaming, bone grafting, and augmented glenoid implants.

Corrective reaming

In the setting of posterior humeral head subluxation with acquired asymmetric posterior glenoid bone loss, a common technique to achieve correction of glenoid retroversion is corrective eccentric reaming. Also referred to as high-side reaming, the surgeon prepares the glenoid in such a way that the anterior glenoid is preferentially reamed to the level of the posterior glenoid surface, thus correcting glenoid version and theoretically recentering the humeral head in a B2 glenoid. However, excessive eccentric reaming results in inadequate bony support for the glenoid implant and can cause joint-line medialization.

Several computer simulation and cadaveric studies have been performed in efforts to define the safe limits of corrective reaming without glenoid vault perforation. Clavert and colleagues[31] conducted a cadaveric study of 5 specimens in which posterior glenoid bone was measured on CT scans. Corrective reaming was then performed guided by a cannulated positioning goniometer set at the measured angle. A pegged glenoid implant with 4 pegs in an inverted T configuration was then implanted. A second CT scan confirmed correction to neutral and assessed fit of the glenoid implant. The mean retroversion created in this study was 24°, and, in all cases, correction to neutral was achieved. The investigators showed peripheral peg penetration and fracture of the anterior glenoid rim as potential complications when performing corrective reaming in deformities exceeding 20° of retroversion.

Nowak and colleagues[32] simulated glenoid resurfacing on 3D models created from CT scans of 19 arthritic shoulders with a mean retroversion of 14.7°. Virtual eccentric reaming to neutral was performed followed by implantation of 3 different sizes of a glenoid component with 3 in-line pegs using computer simulation software. Findings from this study showed that, in all 5 of the 19 patients with preoperative retroversion greater than 18°, no glenoid implant could be implanted without peg penetration at neutral version. Furthermore, 6 of 8 patients that had preoperative retroversion between 12° and 18° were noted to have vault violation when corrected to neutral version with glenoid implants. The investigators also showed that, in challenging cases with severe glenoid retroversion, by downsizing the glenoid component, implantation in less residual retroversion can be achieved with an in-line, pegged component.

Chen and colleagues[33] also recently studied the outcomes of eccentric reaming in a computer simulation study using 25 CT-reconstructed 3D shoulder models of B2 morphology. Virtual TSA was performed with version corrections of 0°, 5°, 10°, and 15°, and density of the bone under the reamed glenoid surface at several depths was measured. They also quantified the remaining high-quality bone after reaming on spatial distribution maps. Findings from this study showed that larger version correction resulted in more bone resection, with poorer remaining bone quality and quantity to support the glenoid implant.

Aleem and colleagues[34] reported a high risk of perforation during corrective reaming of B2 glenoids using a computer simulation model for anatomic TSA. Seventy-one shoulders identified with a B2 glenoid that had preoperative CT scans were included. Virtual implantation of inverted triangle peg or keeled anatomic glenoid implants was performed using 3D computer software, with planned correction to either 15° or 10° of glenoid retroversion. In order to obtain at least 80% implant seating, correction to 15° of retroversion required a mean of 5 mm of reaming, whereas correction to 10° of retroversion required 8 mm of reaming. Corrective reaming to 15° resulted in peripheral peg perforation in 56% of glenoids with greater than 25° of retroversion compared with 23% of glenoids with less than 25° of retroversion. A glenoid with higher native retroversion also was shown to be associated with poor bone quality support when corrected to 15°. The investigators suggested that eccentric reaming may not be ideal in cases of excessive glenoid retroversion and alternative options should be considered.

Although peg perforation is a potential complication of eccentric reaming in excessively retroverted glenoids, clinical outcomes after using this technique at the time of TSA are promising. Gerber and colleagues[35] reported the results of partial corrective reaming at the time of TSA in 23 shoulders found to have a subluxation index of at least 65% as measured on preoperative CT scan. The mean preoperative glenoid retroversion was 18°. Glenoid retroversion was corrected using a glenoid alignment device to a mean retroversion of 9°, not exceeding 15° of correction. Furthermore, posterior subluxation was corrected in 21 of 23 shoulders, and favorable clinical outcomes were reported at a mean follow-up of 3.5 years.

More recently, Orvets and colleagues[36] reported their short-term radiographic and clinical outcomes with TSA after partial corrective reaming in 59 patients with B2 glenoid deformity. The mean preoperative version was 18°, superior inclination was 8°, and posterior subluxation was 67%. At a mean follow-up of 4.2 years, they reported significantly improved clinical outcome scores. At a mean of 2.7 years, radiographic outcomes showed no cases of instability or significant posterior subluxation, and a low risk of progressive glenoid lucencies and implant loosening. Furthermore, no difference with respect to the rate of progression of glenoid radiolucencies was noted in shoulder with less than or equal to 20° compared with those with greater than 20° of retroversion.

Based on the current available literature, eccentric reaming in surgical management of the B2 glenoid is an effective technique in glenoid preparation at the time of TSA to achieve correction of glenoid retroversion and recenter the humeral head. However, the technique should be used judiciously in cases of excessive glenoid retroversion (ie, >15°) to minimize the risk of perforation or anterior glenoid fracture.

Bone grafting

Posterior bone grafting is also a useful adjunct when performing anatomic TSA for B2 glenoids, using either autograft or allograft. This technique is intended to achieve glenoid version correction and enhance bone stock. However, clinical outcome studies after posterior bone grafting have shown varying results.

Neer and Morrison[37] studied 19 shoulders in 18 patients with glenohumeral arthritis of various causes that underwent anatomic TSA augmented with bone graft. They reported 16 excellent outcomes (84%) and 1 satisfactory outcome (5%) at a mean follow-up of 4.4 years. Two patients (11%) were in the limited-goals category. Radiographic analysis showed incomplete radiolucent lines in 6 cases (32%) and no radiolucencies in 13 cases (68%). Their findings supported the role of bone graft augmentation to enhance osseous support of the glenoid component.

Similarly, Steinmann and Cofield[38] published their outcomes after humeral head bone grafting at the time of anatomic TSA in 28 patients, with 19 of those identified as primary osteoarthritis. Several types of glenoid implants were used, including cemented and uncemented. Improved range of motion was observed in all shoulders at a mean follow-up of 5.25 years, with 13 excellent (46%), 10 satisfactory (36%), and 5 (18%) unsatisfactory outcomes. Radiographic analysis revealed the presence of radiolucency in 15 shoulders (54%), 3 of which had a loose glenoid implant. However, symptoms were reported in only 2 of the 3 radiographically loose glenoid implants. Findings from this study showed that bone grafting is a feasible technique to restore glenoid bone stock and correct joint position.

In another study reporting acceptable clinical outcomes after bone grafting, Sabesan and colleagues[39] studied 12 patients with severe glenoid retroversion (mean glenoid retroversion of 44°) treated with autogenous bone grafting at the time of anatomic total shoulder reconstruction. At a mean follow-up of 4.4 years, the investigators reported significant improvement in range of motion postoperatively with an excellent or good clinical outcome based on Penn scores in 10 patients (83%). Complications associated with graft healing and fixation necessitating revision surgery were observed in 2 of 12 patients (17%). These results corroborated findings from prior studies and supported bone grafting to achieve clinical and radiographic improvement in patients with acquired glenoid retroversion, and confirmed the potential for graft-related complications.

Favorable outcomes of bone grafting with longer-term follow-up were reported by Klika and colleagues[40] in 25 shoulders, of which 12 were identified as B2 glenoids. At a mean follow-up of 8.7 years, excellent outcomes were reported in 8 cases and satisfactory outcomes in 2 cases. Aseptic glenoid loosening was observed in 2 shoulders that required revision surgery and had an unsatisfactory outcome. Graft resorption or lack of incorporation was noted in 5 of the 12 B2 glenoids (42%), all of which had excellent outcomes clinically.

Most recently, Nicholson and colleagues[41] studied 28 patients who underwent posterior glenoid bone grafting at the time of anatomic TSA, 13 of which were B1 glenoids and 15 B2 glenoids. The mean glenoid retroversion was 28°. They reported favorable radiographic and clinical outcomes at a mean follow-up of 4 years with significant correction of glenoid retroversion and humeral head subluxation, and improvement in pain, range of motion, and functional outcome scores. Notably, 100% graft incorporation was reported without the need for revision surgery. Hardware complications (broken screws) were reported in 3 patients without any functional impact.

A higher rate of complications associated with bone grafting has been reported by Walch and colleagues[42] who studied outcomes after anatomic TSA in 92 B2 glenoids with a mean intermediate glenoid version of 19°. Posterior glenoid bone grafting was required in 7 shoulders (7.6%) based on preoperative planning because of inability to achieve adequate glenoid retroversion correction (to <10°) with anterior corrective reaming alone. Shoulders requiring bone grafting were associated with significantly worse clinical and radiographic outcomes with respect to active elevation, Constant score, mobility, strength, and radiolucent lines. Glenoid migration after bone graft collapse was reported in 2 cases, but these patients declined revision surgery. Posterior dislocation occurred in 3 shoulders. The investigators cautioned against the use of posterior bone grafting for B2 glenoids given the high rate of complications and inferior clinical outcomes.

Bone graft augmentation is a useful adjunct to TSA to address the acquired glenoid retroversion and posterior glenoid bone loss that is observed in the B2 glenoid. However, it is a technically challenging technique that can be associated with graft-related complications that may affect implant longevity and functional outcome.

Augmented glenoid implants

In an effort to maximize implant stability and minimize the anterior glenoid bone removal needed for seating of the glenoid implant, and to forego the potential complications associated with bone grafting, the use of posteriorly augmented glenoid implants has gained recent popularity. This technique theoretically allows for the preservation of glenoid bone stock and minimizes medialization. Glenoid augments are manufactured in various backside geometries including posterior step, posterior hemiwedge, and full wedge. They can be made of metal or polyethylene.

Several biomechanical studies have evaluated the role of augmented glenoid implants for excessive glenoid retroversion. Iannotti and colleagues[43] reported the results of their in vitro biomechanical study in which 4 different augmented glenoid designs (full wedge with asymmetric spherical backside, full wedge with symmetric spherical backside, full wedge with flat angled backside, and stepped) were compared with a standard anchor peg glenoid. They observed the least anterior component liftoff and superior fixation with a stepped implant in the presence of eccentric loading.

Wang and colleagues[44] biomechanically compared the use of eccentric reaming and standard glenoid placement with the use of augmented glenoid components to address retroversion caused by posterior glenoid bone loss in composite scapula models. They showed increased implant edge displacement and a lower number of specimens reaching the final cycle count without catastrophic failure in the augment group. The investigators suggested that the angled backside geometry of the augment may convert axial load to shear stress at the implant-bone surface leading to micromotion and acceleration of implant loosening. Although the investigators concluded that eccentric reaming with a standard glenoid

component may be biomechanically superior, only incomplete version correction was achieved in the augmented group. In addition, cyclical loading in this study did not include rotation, abduction, or adduction, which also occur with physiologic shoulder movement.

More recently, Sowa and colleagues[45] conducted a biomechanical study to evaluate the effects of various treatment strategies on glenoid component stability in a type B2 glenoid composite scapula model with 15° of glenoid retroversion. Comparison of scapulae treated with eccentric reaming and standard glenoid implantation and half-wedged augmented glenoid at 10,000 cycles showed significantly greater micromotion in the augmented group. Nonetheless, the investigators supported the use of posteriorly augmented glenoids as an alternative strategy to eccentric reaming because it enables retroversion correction while preserving glenoid bone.

Computer modeling studies have also been performed to describe the use of augmented glenoid implants in TSA. Hermida and colleagues[46] performed a finite element analysis comparing standard glenoid implants and full-wedged augments to assess the stresses and strains in the bone, cement, and glenoid components. They reported that the use of a full-wedged glenoid component to correct retroversion significantly decreased stresses and predicted greater bone fatigue life compared with a standard pegged implant. In a 3D computer surgical simulation of 29 patients with glenohumeral osteoarthritis with acquired bone loss and increased retroversion, Sabesan and colleagues[47] showed that glenoid augments can allow complete version correction while minimizing medialization, compared with standard glenoid implants. Kersten and colleagues[48] conducted a similar investigation with virtual implantation of standard, stepped, and wedged components in 10 B2 glenoids and assessed the volume of surgical removal, maximum reaming depth, and percentage of implant surface in contact with cancellous versus cortical bone. The investigators concluded that stepped and wedged augmented glenoid implants both allowed version correction to neutral but required less bone removal and reaming depth, and were supported by more cortical bone compared with standard glenoid implants. These findings were corroborated by a finite element analysis by Allred and colleagues.[49] Furthermore, Knowles and colleagues[50] compared full-wedge, posterior-wedge, and stepped-augment designs in a virtual implantation study of 16 patients with B2 glenoids to assess variations in volume of bone removal and quality of the remaining bone after glenoid preparation. Use of the posterior-wedge design, when correcting to 0°, was shown to require less glenoid bone removal and resulted in superior bone quality of the remaining bone compared with other designs.

There is a paucity of clinical outcomes data on augmented glenoid implants. Such studies have low levels of evidence, small sample sizes, and limited follow-up. Rice and colleagues[51] described their early experience with the use of posterior augments in 14 shoulders of 13 patients and noted marginal benefit. Youderian and colleagues[52] reported good short-term outcomes of a stepped implant in 24 patients undergoing anatomic TSA for severe posterior bone loss with a minimum of 6-month follow-up. Excellent glenoid version correction (mean, 16.7°) with minimal bone loss (mean, 0.45 mm) of the premorbid joint line was noted on postoperative CT scans. In a case-control study, Wright and colleagues[53] reported outcomes in 24 patients with glenohumeral arthritis and posterior glenoid wear treated with anatomic TSA using a full-wedge augment with a minimum of 2-year follow-up. The patients were matched for age, sex, and follow-up to patients without glenoid wear treated with a standard all-polyethylene glenoid. No difference in clinical outcome scores was noted between the two groups but a higher incidence of lucent lines was noted in the augment group. Favorito and colleagues[54] retrospectively assessed clinical outcomes in 22 shoulders with posterior glenoid bone loss treated with an all-polyethylene stepped augment with a mean follow-up of 3 years. A significant improvement in pain, functional scores, and range of motion was noted postoperatively. Osseous integration at the central peg flange was observed in 12 shoulders, and osteolysis occurred in only 1 shoulder. Complications included 2 anterior dislocations requiring revision surgery with a larger head and a posterior dislocation revised to a RTSA. Similarly, Stephens and colleagues[55] described their experience using an all-polyethylene stepped augment in 21 patients with glenohumeral arthritis and a mean retroversion of 20.8° (19 type B2 glenoids, 2 type C glenoids) with a minimum of 2-year follow-up. A significant improvement in pain, motion, functional outcomes, and radiographic parameters was noted. No complications were reported. Radiolucencies around the glenoid were observed in 5 of 21 patients (grade 1 in 4 shoulders, grade 2 in 1 shoulder).

Bony ingrowth around the central peg was observed in 95% of implants, with only 1 shoulder with osteolysis around the central peg. Most recently, Ho and colleagues[56] reported clinical and radiographic outcomes on 71 arthritic shoulders with a B2 or B3 glenoid morphology that underwent anatomic TSA with a stepped augment with a median follow-up of 2.4 years. Range of motion, functional scores, humeral head centering, and glenoid version were all significantly improved postoperatively, and no revision surgery was required. Central peg osteolysis occurred in 11 of 71 shoulders (15%) and was associated with a greater preoperative joint-line medialization and posterior glenoid bone loss compared with those without osteolysis. The investigators suggested that such cases with severe preoperative bone loss, retroversion, and humeral head subluxation may have been better addressed with an RTSA.

The current literature supporting the management of B2 glenoids with augmented glenoid implants consists of biomechanical data, computer modeling studies, and early clinical outcome reports, and is promising. However, longer-term clinical studies with higher levels of evidence will be necessary to define the role of such implants in surgically treating B2 glenoids.

Reverse Total Shoulder Arthroplasty

In certain circumstances, particularly in cases of excessive glenoid retroversion and posterior bone loss with concomitant humeral head subluxation, glenoid reconstruction with TSA can be a challenging endeavor. Walsh and colleagues[42] noted a 44% risk of glenoid loosening when preoperative neoglenoid retroversion exceeded 27° and 11% risk of postoperative posterior humeral head instability when there was greater than 80% humeral head subluxation preoperatively. In addition, there is a heightened risk of peg perforation and inability to restore the native joint line even with eccentric reaming, augmented glenoid implants, or bone grafting. There is a recent trend to treat such challenging cases with reverse shoulder arthroplasty (RSA) with or without posterior glenoid bone grafting. The RTSA confers a semiconstrained design, serving as a potential solution to posterior humeral head subluxation noted in B2 glenoids. Although RTSA is commonly indicated for glenohumeral arthritis in rotator cuff–deficient shoulders, several studies have supported its role in the management the B2 glenoid despite the presence of an intact rotator cuff.

Mizuno and colleagues[57] evaluated the clinical and radiographic outcomes of RTSA for biconcave glenoids with primary osteoarthritis without the presence of rotator cuff insufficiency. The mean preoperative retroversion was 32°, and mean humeral head subluxation was 87% as evaluated using CT. In 27 shoulders with a mean follow-up of 4.5 years, the investigators reported a significant increase in Constant scores, strength, pain, range of motion in all planes, and activities of daily living after RSA. Although no radiolucent lines were observed around the central peg or baseplate screws, scapular notching was noted in 10 shoulders (37%). Recurrence of posterior humeral head instability was not reported. Neurologic complications occurred in 3 patients. Of the 10 patients that underwent bone graft augmentation, 1 patient experienced early loosening of the glenoid component.

McFarland and colleagues[58] also reported on the use of RTSA to treat glenohumeral arthritis in cuff-intact shoulders. In 42 consecutive patients, RTSA was performed after reaming the glenoid flat such that there was a congruent surface between the bone and glenoid component. Patients in this study included 19 A2 glenoids, 5 B2 glenoids, and 18 C glenoids. The mean retroversions were 10.9°, 17.5°, and 31.9° for A2, B2, and C glenoids respectively. Results showed improved pain and functional outcomes postoperatively. With respect to range of motion, significant postoperative improvement was noted in active abduction, flexion, and external rotation with the arm elevated 90°. In addition, improvement with active external rotation with the arm at the side and active internal rotation with the arm elevated to 90° was observed but did not reach statistical significance. Radiographically, the investigators reported scapular notching in 8 shoulders (19%), occurring in 3 of the 5 cases noted to have B2 glenoid morphology. Baseplate failure occurred in 1 patient with a type C glenoid that required revision with bone grafting. The investigators showed a favorable clinical outcome with RTSA for treatment of osteoarthritis and glenoid bone loss in shoulders with a functional rotator cuff.

Bone graft augmentation while performing RTSA for osteoarthritis has also been reported. Lorenzetti and colleagues[59] studied their outcomes after bone graft augmentation for severe glenoid bone in primary RTSA in 57 patients. Humeral head autograft (52 shoulders) or femoral head autograft (5 shoulders) was placed as described by Klein and colleagues.[60] In addition to clinical outcomes, they determined the exact position of the implants postoperatively using 3D reconstructions of preoperative CT scans combined with postoperative radiographs at 3 months by using contour projection shape-mapping algorithms, allowing them to further assess native bone support. At a mean follow-up of 3.8 years, the investigators reported significant improvement in pain, function, and range of motion all planes and a 98% rate of full graft incorporation. No cases of glenoid baseplate failure were observed. Furthermore, the mean percentage of the implant supported by native bone was 17% (range, 0%–50%), and the functional outcome was not related to the degree of native bone supporting the glenoid implant. Although rotator cuff arthropathy constituted most cases (38 shoulders), and only 7 patients were identified with primary glenohumeral osteoarthritis (3 A2 glenoids, 2 B2 glenoids, and 2 C glenoids), the results of this study suggest a role of RTSA and bone graft augmentation in treating shoulders with severe bone loss.

Boileau and colleagues[61] reported on the use of an angled biologic increased-offset RTSA grafting technique in 54 patients undergoing RTSA for various disorders, including advanced glenohumeral arthritis and rotator cuff arthropathy. They described using a trapezoid humeral head autograft to correct version and/or inclination. Fifteen B2 glenoids were included. The investigators reported the enhanced ability to correct glenoid version and superior inclination with the described technique, with a 94% graft incorporation rate and significant improvement in postoperative range of motion and functional scores.

Harmsen and colleagues[62] described the radiographic and functional outcomes of a shaped humeral head autograft for RTSA for shoulders with significant posterior glenoid bone loss but an intact rotator cuff. In their study of 29 shoulders with 16 B2 glenoids, 10 B3 glenoids, and 3 C glenoids, the mean preoperative glenoid retroversion was 32.3°. In preparing the glenoid using a cannulated system, the anterior glenoid was eccentrically reamed to the guidewire, and the posterior glenoid was trephinated and decorticated. Humeral head autografts were shaped such that the anterior portion of the graft was perpendicular to the reamed glenoid and the posterior portion of the graft matched the neoglenoid version. The autograft was secured to the glenoid using a long post baseplate along with a combination of 2 peripheral compression screws and 2 peripheral locking screws. At a mean follow-up of 2.8 years, range of motion, strength, and functional outcome scores improved significantly compared with preoperatively. Graft incorporation was noted in all cases radiographically. Recurrent instability and glenoid baseplate fixation failure were not observed. Infection was present in 2 cases, 1 being superficial and subsequently managed with oral antibiotics and the deep infection requiring a 2-stage revision. At the time of revision surgery, the graft had fully healed and there was no evidence of baseplate loosening. This study strongly supported a role of bone graft augmentation in B2 glenoids undergoing RTSA.

Keener and colleagues[63] described the optimal humeral and glenoid component position in patients with primary glenohumeral osteoarthritis with severe glenoid retroversion deformity. In their computer simulation study, 10 shoulders identified as B2, B3, or C deformities with glenoid retroversion exceeding 25° and posterior humeral subluxation greater than 80% were planned for RTSA. Using preoperative CT scans and 3D templating software, the glenoid was implanted with varying reaming depths, degrees of retroversion, and lateral offset, and a short-stemmed onlay humeral component was placed with varying angles of inclination. After planning the desired glenoid and humeral component positions, a range-of-motion analysis was performed using automated software. Optimal postimplantation range of motion was achieved with a glenoid implant having 10 mm of baseplate lateralization with neutral to 5° of retroversion and 135° angle of inclination on the humeral implant.

RTSA is gaining popularity to alleviate pain and restore function in patients with challenging shoulder disorders such as the B2 glenoid deformity. As indications for RTSA continue to expand, its role in managing the biconcave glenoid with excessive retroversion will continue to be defined with longer-term studies assessing functional and radiographic outcomes. In addition, augmented baseplates are becoming available to help fill in bony defects, and show early promising results.

SUMMARY

Management of the B2 glenoid for primary osteoarthritis of the glenohumeral joint remains a challenge. Arthroscopic debridement does not provide long-term durable results. With regard to arthroplasty, there are several relative advantages and disadvantages to the techniques described. Surgeons must consider patient-specific factors and the overall deformity in the shoulder to tailor appropriate arthroplasty treatment.

REFERENCES

1. Neer CS 2nd. Replacement arthroplasty for glenohumeral osteoarthritis. J Bone Joint Surg Am 1974; 56(1):1–13.
2. Neer CS 2nd, Watson KC, Stanton FJ. Recent experience in total shoulder replacement. J Bone Joint Surg Am 1982;64(3):319–37.
3. Walch G, Badet R, Boulahia A, et al. Morphologic study of the glenoid in primary glenohumeral osteoarthritis. J Arthroplasty 1999;14(6):756–60.
4. Bercik MJ, Kruse K 2nd, Yalizis M, et al. A modification to the Walch classification of the glenoid in primary glenohumeral osteoarthritis using three-dimensional imaging. J Shoulder Elbow Surg 2016;25(10):1601–6.
5. Beuckelaers E, Jacxsens M, Van Tongel A, et al. Three-dimensional computed tomography scan evaluation of the pattern of erosion in type B glenoids. J Shoulder Elbow Surg 2014;23(1):109–16.
6. Hoenecke HR Jr, Tibor LM, D'Lima DD. Glenoid morphology rather than version predicts humeral subluxation: a different perspective on the glenoid in total shoulder arthroplasty. J Shoulder Elbow Surg 2012;21(9):1136–41.
7. Churchill RS, Spencer EE Jr, Fehringer EV. Quantification of B2 glenoid morphology in total shoulder arthroplasty. J Shoulder Elbow Surg 2015;24(8): 1212–7.
8. Domos P, Checchia CS, Walch G. Walch B0 glenoid: pre-osteoarthritic posterior subluxation of the humeral head. J Shoulder Elbow Surg 2018; 27(1):181–8.
9. Friedman RJ, Hawthorne KB, Genez BM. The use of computerized tomography in the measurement of glenoid version. J Bone Joint Surg Am 1992;74(7): 1032–7.
10. Rouleau DM, Kidder JF, Pons-Villanueva J, et al. Glenoid version: how to measure it? Validity of different methods in two-dimensional computed tomography scans. J Shoulder Elbow Surg 2010; 19(8):1230–7.
11. Walch G, Ascani C, Boulahia A, et al. Static posterior subluxation of the humeral head: an unrecognized entity responsible for glenohumeral osteoarthritis in the young adult. J Shoulder Elbow Surg 2002;11(4):309–14.
12. Kidder J, Rouleau D, Pons-Villanueva J, et al. Humeral head posterior subluxation on CT scan: validation and comparison of 2 methods of measurement. Tech Shoulder Elbow Surg 2010; 11(3):72–6.
13. Kerr BJ, McCarty EC. Outcome of arthroscopic debridement is worse for patients with

glenohumeral arthritis of both sides of the joint. Clin Orthop Relat Res 2008;466(3):634–8.

14. Richards DP, Burkhart SS. Arthroscopic debridement and capsular release for glenohumeral osteoarthritis. Arthroscopy 2007;23(9):1019–22.

15. Spiegl UJ, Faucett SC, Horan MP, et al. The role of arthroscopy in the management of glenohumeral osteoarthritis: a Markov decision model. Arthroscopy 2014;30(11):1392–9.

16. Mitchell JJ, Horan MP, Greenspoon JA, et al. Survivorship and patient-reported outcomes after comprehensive arthroscopic management of glenohumeral osteoarthritis: minimum 5-year follow-up. Am J Sports Med 2016;44(12):3206–13.

17. Mitchell JJ, Warner BT, Horan MP, et al. Comprehensive arthroscopic management of glenohumeral osteoarthritis: preoperative factors predictive of treatment failure. Am J Sports Med 2017;45(4): 794–802.

18. Millett PJ, Fritz EM, Frangiamore SJ, et al. Arthroscopic management of glenohumeral arthritis: a joint preservation approach. J Am Acad Orthop Surg 2018;26(21):745–52.

19. Cameron BD, Galatz LM, Ramsey ML, et al. Nonprosthetic management of grade IV osteochondral lesions of the glenohumeral joint. J Shoulder Elbow Surg 2002;11(1):25–32.

20. de Beer JF, Bhatia DN, van Rooyen KS, et al. Arthroscopic debridement and biological resurfacing of the glenoid in glenohumeral arthritis. Knee Surg Sports Traumatol Arthrosc 2010;18(12): 1767–73.

21. Van Thiel GS, Sheehan S, Frank RM, et al. Retrospective analysis of arthroscopic management of glenohumeral degenerative disease. Arthroscopy 2010;26(11):1451–5.

22. Millett PJ, Gaskill TR. Arthroscopic trans-capsular axillary nerve decompression: indication and surgical technique. Arthroscopy 2011;27(10):1444–8.

23. Millett PJ, Horan MP, Pennock AT, et al. Comprehensive Arthroscopic Management (CAM) procedure: clinical results of a joint-preserving arthroscopic treatment for young, active patients with advanced shoulder osteoarthritis. Arthroscopy 2013;29(3):440–8.

24. Mook WR, Petri M, Greenspoon JA, et al. The comprehensive arthroscopic management procedure for treatment of glenohumeral osteoarthritis. Arthrosc Tech 2015;4(5):e435–41.

25. Levine WN, Djurasovic M, Glasson JM, et al. Hemiarthroplasty for glenohumeral osteoarthritis: results correlated to degree of glenoid wear. J Shoulder Elbow Surg 1997;6(5):449–54.

26. Levine WN, Fischer CR, Nguyen D, et al. Long-term follow-up of shoulder hemiarthroplasty for glenohumeral osteoarthritis. J Bone Joint Surg Am 2012;94(22):e164.

27. Matsen FA 3rd. The ream and run: not for every patient, every surgeon or every problem. International orthopaedics 2015;39:255–61.

28. Lynch JR, Franta AK, Montgomery WH Jr, et al. Self-assessed outcome at two to four years after shoulder hemiarthroplasty with concentric glenoid reaming. J Bone Joint Surg Am 2007;89(6):1284–92.

29. Gilmer BB, Comstock BA, Jette JL, et al. The prognosis for improvement in comfort and function after the ream-and-run arthroplasty for glenohumeral arthritis: an analysis of 176 consecutive cases. J Bone Joint Surg Am 2012;94(14):e102.

30. Weldon EJ 3rd, Boorman RS, Smith KL, et al. Optimizing the glenoid contribution to the stability of a humeral hemiarthroplasty without a prosthetic glenoid. J Bone Joint Surg Am 2004;86-A(9):2022–9.

31. Clavert P, Millett PJ, Warner JJ. Glenoid resurfacing: what are the limits to asymmetric reaming for posterior erosion? J Shoulder Elbow Surg 2007; 16(6):843–8.

32. Nowak DD, Bahu MJ, Gardner TR, et al. Simulation of surgical glenoid resurfacing using three-dimensional computed tomography of the arthritic glenohumeral joint: the amount of glenoid retroversion that can be corrected. J Shoulder Elbow Surg 2009;18(5):680–8.

33. Chen X, Reddy AS, Kontaxis A, et al. Version correction via eccentric reaming compromises remaining bone quality in B2 glenoids: a computational study. Clin Orthop Relat Res 2017;475(12):3090–9.

34. Aleem AW, Orvets ND, Patterson BC, et al. Risk of perforation is high during corrective reaming of retroverted glenoids: a computer simulation study. Clin Orthop Relat Res 2018;476(8):1612–9.

35. Gerber C, Costouros JG, Sukthankar A, et al. Static posterior humeral head subluxation and total shoulder arthroplasty. J Shoulder Elbow Surg 2009;18(4):505–10.

36. Orvets ND, Chamberlain AM, Patterson BM, et al. Total shoulder arthroplasty in patients with a B2 glenoid addressed with corrective reaming. J Shoulder Elbow Surg 2018;27(6S):S58–64.

37. Neer CS 2nd, Morrison DS. Glenoid bone-grafting in total shoulder arthroplasty. J Bone Joint Surg Am 1988;70(8):1154–62.

38. Steinmann SP, Cofield RH. Bone grafting for glenoid deficiency in total shoulder replacement. J Shoulder Elbow Surg 2000;9(5):361–7.

39. Sabesan V, Callanan M, Ho J, et al. Clinical and radiographic outcomes of total shoulder arthroplasty with bone graft for osteoarthritis with severe glenoid bone loss. J Bone Joint Surg Am 2013; 95(14):1290–6.

40. Klika BJ, Wooten CW, Sperling JW, et al. Structural bone grafting for glenoid deficiency in primary total shoulder arthroplasty. J Shoulder Elbow Surg 2014;23(7):1066–72.

41. Nicholson GP, Cvetanovich GL, Rao AJ, et al. Posterior glenoid bone grafting in total shoulder arthroplasty for osteoarthritis with severe posterior glenoid wear. J Shoulder Elbow Surg 2017;26(10):1844–53.

42. Walch G, Moraga C, Young A, et al. Results of anatomic nonconstrained prosthesis in primary osteoarthritis with biconcave glenoid. J Shoulder Elbow Surg 2012;21(11):1526–33.

43. Iannotti JP, Lappin KE, Klotz CL, et al. Liftoff resistance of augmented glenoid components during cyclic fatigue loading in the posterior-superior direction. J Shoulder Elbow Surg 2013;22(11):1530–6.

44. Wang T, Abrams GD, Behn AW, et al. Posterior glenoid wear in total shoulder arthroplasty: eccentric anterior reaming is superior to posterior augment. Clin Orthop Relat Res 2015;473(12):3928–36.

45. Sowa B, Bochenek M, Braun S, et al. Replacement options for the B2 glenoid in osteoarthritis of the shoulder: a biomechanical study. Arch Orthop Trauma Surg 2018;138(7):891–9.

46. Hermida JC, Flores-Hernandez C, Hoenecke HR, et al. Augmented wedge-shaped glenoid component for the correction of glenoid retroversion: a finite element analysis. J Shoulder Elbow Surg 2014;23(3):347–54.

47. Sabesan V, Callanan M, Sharma V, et al. Correction of acquired glenoid bone loss in osteoarthritis with a standard versus an augmented glenoid component. J Shoulder Elbow Surg 2014;23(7):964–73.

48. Kersten AD, Flores-Hernandez C, Hoenecke HR, et al. Posterior augmented glenoid designs preserve more bone in biconcave glenoids. J Shoulder Elbow Surg 2015;24(7):1135–41.

49. Allred JJ, Flores-Hernandez C, Hoenecke HR Jr, et al. Posterior augmented glenoid implants require less bone removal and generate lower stresses: a finite element analysis. J Shoulder Elbow Surg 2016;25(5):823–30.

50. Knowles NK, Ferreira LM, Athwal GS. Augmented glenoid component designs for type B2 erosions: a computational comparison by volume of bone removal and quality of remaining bone. J Shoulder Elbow Surg 2015;24(8):1218–26.

51. Rice RS, Sperling JW, Miletti J, et al. Augmented glenoid component for bone deficiency in shoulder arthroplasty. Clin Orthop Relat Res 2008;466(3):579–83.

52. Youderian A, Napolitano L A, Davidson I, et al. Management of glenoid bone loss with the use of a new augmented all-polyethylene glenoid component. Tech Shoulder Elbow Surg 2012;13(4):163–9.

53. Wright TW, Grey SG, Roche CP, et al. Preliminary results of a posterior augmented glenoid compared to an all polyethylene standard glenoid in anatomic total shoulder arthroplasty. Bull Hosp Jt Dis (2013) 2015;73(Suppl 1):S79–85.

54. Favorito PJ, Freed RJ, Passanise AM, et al. Total shoulder arthroplasty for glenohumeral arthritis associated with posterior glenoid bone loss: results of an all-polyethylene, posteriorly augmented glenoid component. J Shoulder Elbow Surg 2016;25(10):1681–9.

55. Stephens SP, Spencer EE, Wirth MA. Radiographic results of augmented all-polyethylene glenoids in the presence of posterior glenoid bone loss during total shoulder arthroplasty. J Shoulder Elbow Surg 2017;26(5):798–803.

56. Ho JC, Amini MH, Entezari V, et al. Clinical and radiographic outcomes of a posteriorly augmented glenoid component in anatomic total shoulder arthroplasty for primary osteoarthritis with posterior glenoid bone loss. J Bone Joint Surg Am 2018;100(22):1934–48.

57. Mizuno N, Denard PJ, Raiss P, et al. Reverse total shoulder arthroplasty for primary glenohumeral osteoarthritis in patients with a biconcave glenoid. J Bone Joint Surg Am 2013;95(14):1297–304.

58. McFarland EG, Huri G, Hyun YS, et al. Reverse total shoulder arthroplasty without bone-grafting for severe glenoid bone loss in patients with osteoarthritis and intact rotator cuff. J Bone Joint Surg Am 2016;98(21):1801–7.

59. Lorenzetti A, Streit JJ, Cabezas AF, et al. Bone graft augmentation for severe glenoid bone loss in primary reverse total shoulder arthroplasty: outcomes and evaluation of host bone contact by 2D-3D image registration. JB JS Open Access 2017;2(3):e0015.

60. Klein SM, Dunning P, Mulieri P, et al. Effects of acquired glenoid bone defects on surgical technique and clinical outcomes in reverse shoulder arthroplasty. The Journal of bone and joint surgery American volume 2010;92:1144–54.

61. Boileau P, Morin-Salvo N, Gauci MO, et al. Angled BIO-RSA (bony-increased offset-reverse shoulder arthroplasty): a solution for the management of glenoid bone loss and erosion. J Shoulder Elbow Surg 2017;26(12):2133–42.

62. Harmsen S, Casagrande D, Norris T. "Shaped" humeral head autograft reverse shoulder arthroplasty: Treatment for primary glenohumeral osteoarthritis with significant posterior glenoid bone loss (B2, B3, and C type). Orthopade 2017;46(12):1045–54.

63. Keener JD, Patterson BM, Orvets N, et al. Optimizing reverse shoulder arthroplasty component position in the setting of advanced arthritis with posterior glenoid erosion: a computer-enhanced range of motion analysis. J Shoulder Elbow Surg 2018;27(2):339–49.

Arthroscopic Management of Glenohumeral Arthritis

David C. Carver, MD[a], Tyler J. Brolin, MD[b],*

KEYWORDS

- Glenohumeral arthritis • Comprehensive arthroscopic management • Chondroplasty
- Microfracture • Humeral osteophyte • Axillary nerve compression

KEY POINTS

- Glenohumeral arthritis in the young adult is a particularly challenging condition for which optimal treatment algorithms have yet to be established.
- Arthroscopic joint-preserving treatments have the advantage of delaying arthroplasty in this younger population while maintaining the patient's natural anatomy and do not appear to compromise later arthroplasty.
- Various surgical techniques are available such that the overall procedure is tailored to the patient's individual pathology.
- Most short- and mid-term studies show good outcomes with low conversion to total shoulder arthroplasty and sustained improvements in functional outcome scores.

INTRODUCTION

Osteoarthritis is the most common cause of disability in the United States.[1] Glenohumeral osteoarthritis (GHOA) is a common cause of shoulder pain and dysfunction leading to decreased range of motion, pain with activity, and sleep disturbance. In particular, GHOA has previously been shown to impact a patient's health similar to other chronic medical conditions, such as congestive heart failure, acute myocardial infarction, diabetes mellitus, and clinical depression.[2]

When nonoperative treatment options have been exhausted including activity restriction, oral anti-inflammatory medication, corticosteroid injections, and potential viscosupplementation, operative treatment is indicated. In the older, less-active patient with a diagnosis of GHOA, total shoulder arthroplasty (TSA) continues to be the mainstay of treatment, as it has previously been shown to provide reliable pain relief and functional improvement.[3–7]

However, the treatment of GHOA in the young patient with greater functional demands is difficult, and the optimal treatment has yet to be established.[8] The outcomes of shoulder arthroplasty in younger patients are inferior to those in older patients, with studies showing that age less than 50 years is a predictor of worse outcomes after shoulder arthroplasty.[9–12] Younger patients undergoing arthroplasty also experience higher rates of component failure.[13] Specifically, in studies investigating long-term (>10 years) outcomes among patients younger than 55 years of age after total shoulder arthroplasty, implant survival ranges between 62.5% and 83.2%.[14,15] Another recent study of total shoulder arthroplasty in patients younger than 65 years showed an overall rate of glenoid lucencies of 54% at a mean follow-up of 9.4 years.[12] There are several reasons younger patients experience worse

Disclosure Statement: The authors have nothing to disclose.
[a] Lake Tahoe Sports Medicine Fellowship, 212 Elks Point Road, Suite 200, PO Box 11889, Zephyr Cove, NV 89448, USA; [b] Department of Orthopaedic Surgery, Campbell Clinic, University of Tennessee Health Science Center, Memphis, TN 38104, USA
* Corresponding author. 1458 West Poplar Avenue, Suite 100, Collierville, TN 38107.
E-mail address: tbrolin@campbellclinic.com
; @carversportsmed (D.C.C.)

outcomes associated with arthroplasty, including: relatively greater impairment of shoulder function preoperatively; different, and sometimes more complex diagnoses; increased demands and activity levels; increased expectations; and increased longevity.[9,16–21]

Hemiarthroplasty has also been used for the treatment of GHOA in younger patients. Theoretically this avoids potential complications associated with glenoid implantation and limitations on postoperative activities. However, long-term studies have shown mixed results. In 1 long-term study of hemiarthroplasty in patients younger than 55 years,[11] 42% of patients were considered to have an unsatisfactory result, and 15-year survivorship was only 73%. A recent systematic review and meta-analysis comparing total shoulder arthroplasty with hemiarthroplasty for the treatment of GHOA in patients younger than age 60 years showed that total shoulder arthroplasty provides greater improvement of pain and range of motion than does hemiarthroplasty. However, patient satisfaction was similar, and revision surgery was equally as likely.[22] Other authors have described hemiarthroplasty with biologic resurfacing of the glenoid, but this is also associated with high failure rates.[23] Additionally, a recent economic decision model showed that total shoulder arthroplasty was more cost-effective compared with hemiarthroplasty in the treatment of GHOA in patients ages 30 to 50 years, as total shoulder arthroplasty is associated with a lower risk of revision in the long term.[24] As a result, outcomes after hemiarthroplasty for GHOA remain guarded in this patient population, given the high revision rates and inferior outcomes compared with total shoulder arthroplasty.

Therefore, younger patients with glenohumeral arthritis pose a significant challenge to the shoulder surgeon. Despite these findings, the demand for shoulder arthroplasty in patients 55 years of age or younger is increasing yearly.[25] Treatment protocols that could potentially delay time to arthroplasty, while still providing improved functional outcomes, would be particularly beneficial to this particular patient population. Recent developments in arthroscopic management have provided the surgeon with nonarthroplasty alternatives in order to obtain clinically meaningful outcomes for this select patient population.

CLINICAL EVALUATION

Clinical evaluation of the young patient with glenohumeral arthritis begins with a detailed history and physical examination. Important questions include the timing of pain (acute vs insidious), history of trauma, history of prior surgical intervention, and interventions that have already been attempted. In regards to prior surgical intervention, patients with instability may have undergone anterior stabilizing procedures resulting in capsulorrhaphy arthropathy. Patients may have been treated with intra-articular pain pumps in the postoperative period, resulting in chondrolysis of the articular cartilage.[26,27] A history of steroid use or alcohol use may indicate avascular necrosis as the underlying etiology. It is also important to evaluate for the diagnosis of inflammatory arthritis, which would preclude arthroscopic management.[17]

Several aspects of the physical examination deserve special attention. Inspection of the skin for surgical incisions can help better understand previous surgical interventions that have been performed and could potentially impact future surgical planning. Areas of warmth and erythema, particularly if around previous surgical incisions, may raise concern for infection and/or septic arthritis. Palpation of the shoulder girdle may indicate acromioclavicular joint disease or tendonitis of the proximal biceps tendon, both of which may need to be addressed surgically. Range-of-motion testing is particularly important, as patients with glenohumeral arthritis commonly have associated limitations in motion that could also be addressed surgically with either a manipulation or capsular release. Strength testing may reveal weakness of particular muscle groups, resulting from compressive neuropathies (axillary nerve, suprascapular nerve) or rotator cuff tears.

Imaging of the glenohumeral joint shoulder includes a series of standard shoulder radiographs to evaluate the glenoid morphology, remaining joint space, osteophyte formation, possible loose body formation, and any deformity that may have developed either from traumatic or developmental etiologies (Fig. 1). The most common bony abnormality encountered in glenohumeral osteoarthritis is the formation of osteophytes along the articular margin of the humeral head and along the line of attachment of the labrum to the glenoid, with as many as 91% of patients showing some degree of humeral head osteophyte formation.[28] Osteophytes in the humeral head are best viewed radiographically during external rotation of the humerus. However, plain films underestimate the degree of osteophyte formation involving both the humeral head and glenoid.[28] Studies

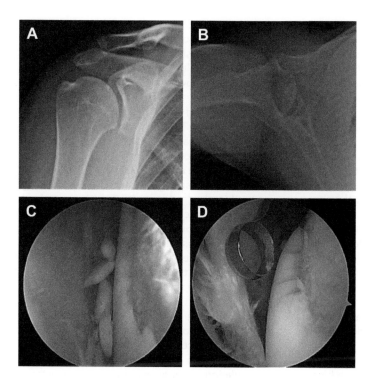

Fig. 1. (A) Grashey and (B) axillary lateral radiographs of a 48-year-old man with chronic right shoulder pain demonstrating a well-preserved glenohumeral joint space and minimal osteophyte formation at the inferior humeral head and inferior glenoid. (C, D) Arthroscopic images as viewed through a posterior viewing portal with the patient in the beach chair position. (C) Extensive grade 4 cartilage loss on the humeral head and multiple loose bodies are visualized. (D) The patient underwent glenohumeral joint debridement with loose body removal and stabilization and contouring of the humeral head articular cartilage, biceps tenodesis, limited capsular release, and subacromial decompression.

have shown that joint space narrowing and osteophyte formation are reliable and independent predictors of primary shoulder arthritis and should be taken into account for clinical decision making.[29]

Advanced imaging is also usually obtained in the form of computed tomography (CT) or MRI to further evaluate the remaining cartilage, the glenoid morphology, and possible loose body formation. MRI, in particular, can provide useful information regarding the degree and location of cartilage lesions (unipolar vs bipolar), status of the rotator cuff, degree of biceps tendon pathology, degree of subcoracoid impingement, and loose body formation.

Last, it is important to understand the patient's goals and expectations and their desired occupation and activity levels. An active patient who desires to continue with competitive sporting events might best be suited with arthroscopic management. Conversely, a sedentary patient with limited physical demands on the upper extremity may best be suited with arthroplasty. It is also important for the patient to fully understand that arthroscopic management is still considered by many to be a palliative treatment option, meant to ultimately delay time to arthroplasty and is not intended to be a definitive treatment for osteoarthritis.

CONSERVATIVE TREATMENT

Nonoperative management of glenohumeral arthritis consists of activity and/or occupation modifications, anti-inflammatory medications, and intra-articular injections.[4,13,30] Physical therapy should be directed at improving range of motion and maintaining strength; however, its utility in GHOA is limited. Non-narcotic pain medicine and intra-articular injections are also commonly used, although with limited evidence.[31] However, if intra-articular injections are used, some authors recommend no more than 3 corticosteroid injections into a single joint unless there are special circumstances.[4] Although nonsurgical management will not alter the long-term disease progression of arthritis, it can be effective in reducing pain and maintaining or even improving range of motion, thereby delaying definitive treatment with arthroplasty.[32]

SURGICAL TREATMENT

The ideal surgical candidate is a younger, active patient with mild-to-moderate osteoarthritis who remains symptomatic despite conservative treatment. A Markov decision analysis showed that arthroscopic management might be better suited for patients younger than 47 years of age, and that total shoulder arthroplasty might be better suited for patients older than 66 years. However, between 47 and 66 years of age there is not a clear advantage of one technique over the other.[33] Inferior outcomes have been reported when there is severe joint incongruity, large osteophytes, and bipolar chondral lesions.[34,35] Outcomes are less predictable and less durable if there are less than 2 mm of glenohumeral joint space remaining.[36] Patients with Kellgren-Lawrence grade 3 or 4 arthritis, or a Walch type B2 or C glenoid are also more likely to experience early failure of arthroscopic management.[37]

Various joint-preserving techniques have been reported for the patient with glenohumeral arthritis. The specific pathology identified on clinical and/or radiographic examination will allow the clinician to discern which techniques will result in improved outcomes for the patient. Generally speaking, the goals of arthroscopic treatment include stabilizing chondral defects, eliminating mechanical crepitation, addressing capsular contracture, addressing known pain generators such as the long head of the biceps, and relieving nerve compression (**Fig. 2**).

Isolated chondral defects can be treated arthroscopically with either debridement alone, or with microfracture in order to generate the production of fibrocartilage over the cartilage defect. Arthroscopic debridement of chondral lesions is carried down to a stable rim of cartilage and subchondral bone. A stable, vertical transition zone should be created at the rim of the defect.[30] Although much of the literature regarding marrow stimulation techniques deals with the knee, the principles remain similar, with the goal of creating a fibrocartilage layer over the defect. The technique for microfracture is similar to that described for the knee by Steadman and colleagues.[38] The lesion should be defined with a stable perpendicular edge of healthy viable cartilage around the defect using a combination of curettes and motorized shavers. The calcified cartilage layer in the base of the defect should be removed using a curette, leaving an exposed layer of subchondral bone. Awls are then used to penetrate the subchondral bone to allow the mesenchymal marrow elements to form a fibrin scaffold, which is eventually replaced by fibrocartilage.[38] Marrow stimulation techniques do not appear to preclude future reconstructive surgeries.[39]

Stiffness, a common finding in this patient population, can be addressed with either a manipulation under anesthesia or with an arthroscopic capsular release. Preoperative physical examination will allow the surgeon to identify which motions are reduced to allow for proper capsular release. A difference of 15 degrees of motion in any plane compared with the contralateral extremity is often used as a guide for

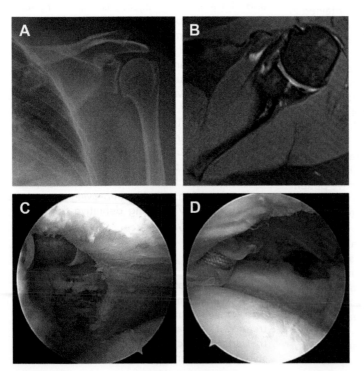

Fig. 2. (A) Grashey radiograph of a 44-year-old man with longstanding left shoulder pain and stiffness demonstrating moderate glenohumeral joint space narrowing and osteophyte formation at the inferior humeral head. (B) MRI demonstrating full-thickness chondral defect on the glenoid with underlying subchondral edema. (C, D) Arthroscopic images as viewed through a posterior viewing portal with the patient in the beach chair position. The patient underwent glenohumeral joint debridement, (C) complete capsular release, (D) biceps tenodesis, and subacromial decompression.

determining the need for arthroscopic capsular release.[40,41]

Biceps tendinopathy can be treated with either tenodesis or tenotomy, although in this typically younger and more active population, tenodesis is the authors' preferred technique. Subacromial impingement can be addressed with subacromial bursectomy and acromioplasty. Acromioclavicular joint arthritis can be treated with either arthroscopic or open distal clavicle excision. Coracoid impingement is often associated with anterior shoulder pain, increased pain with internal rotation, and fraying of the upper border of the subscapularis tendon. Subcoracoid decompression is indicated with these findings, or a subcoracoid distance of less than 7 to 10 mm.[16,42] Various other procedures also can be performed, including loose body removal, synovectomy, and labral debridement if indicated based on clinical examination.

Recently, Millett and colleagues[41] described their comprehensive arthroscopic management (CAM) for glenohumeral arthritis in young adults. The CAM procedure adds inferior humeral osteoplasty and axillary nerve decompression to the previously described techniques of arthroscopic glenohumeral debridement, chondroplasty, synovectomy, loose body removal, capsular releases, subacromial decompression, subcoracoid decompression, and biceps tenodesis/tenotomy when indicated.[40,43,44] Detailed technique descriptions of that technique have been previously reported and are beyond the scope of this article.[40,41,43,44] Indications for axillary nerve decompression include patients with posterior and/or lateral shoulder pain, atrophy of the teres minor or deltoid, external rotation weakness without rotator cuff tear, displacement of the axillary nerve as seen on preoperative MRI, or fatty infiltration of the teres minor as seen on preoperative MRI.[41,43] Previous studies by Millett and colleagues[45] have shown an association between the size of the inferior humeral head osteophyte and fatty infiltration of the teres minor, suggesting a possible etiology for compressive neuropathy of the axillary nerve.

OUTCOMES

Studies support the idea that outcomes are related to the size and location of articular lesions. The first report of arthroscopic management of glenohumeral osteoarthritis was from Ogilvie-Harris and Wiley.[46] Their report of 54 patients with osteoarthritis of the shoulder with mean 3-year follow-up showed good results in two-thirds of patients with mild degeneration,

compared with only one-third of patients with severe degeneration. Patients with a frozen shoulder also seemed to benefit more after having a capsular release and manipulation performed.[46] In a retrospective review of 61 patients with Outerbridge grade 4 cartilage lesions treated with arthroscopic debridement, pain relief was obtained in 88% of patients. The mean duration of pain relief was 28 months. However, articular lesions greater than 2 cm^2 were associated with return of pain and failure of the procedure.[47]

Other more recent studies have shown that arthroscopic debridement can result in significant improvements in functional outcome scores, as well as objective measures of range of motion.[35] Other studies also show that arthroscopic management results in better outcomes when the glenohumeral joint remains concentric and when there is still visible joint space on the axillary radiograph.[34] However, other studies suggest that the size and severity of the lesion is less important than the location. In a retrospective study of 20 shoulders in patients younger than 55 years, Kerr and McCarty[48] found that outcomes were similar for patients with isolated Outerbridge grade 2 and 3 lesions compared with isolated grade 4 lesions. However, patients with bipolar lesions had significantly worse outcomes when compared to patients with unipolar lesions. At less than 2 years follow-up, 3 patients (15%) had progressed to shoulder resurfacing or arthroplasty.[48]

In the first study of the CAM procedure, Millett and colleagues[41] reported the outcomes of 30 shoulders at a minimum of 24 months follow-up. Diffuse Outerbridge grade 4 changes were noted in 21 of the humeral heads and in 20 of the glenoids. The mean American Shoulder and Elbow Surgeons (ASES) score improved from 58 points preoperatively to 83 points postoperatively. Six patients (20%) had progressed to arthroplasty at a mean of 1.9 years postoperatively. Survivorship analysis showed a 92% survival rate at 1 year and 85% at 2 years. A follow-up study from the same group reported minimum 5-year outcomes after the CAM procedure. Of 49 shoulders, 12 (26%) had progressed to total shoulder arthroplasty at a mean of 2.6 years postoperatively. Survivorship analysis showed arthroplasty-free survival of 95.6% at 1 year, 86.7% at 3 years, and 76.9% at 5 years. More encouraging, however, was that for those shoulders that did not progress to arthroplasty, the mean ASES score at 5 years was 85 points, and median patient satisfaction was of 9 out of 10, suggesting that for these patients, arthroscopic management provided a sustained improvement in functional outcome scores.[49]

Several factors have been found to correlate with early failure of the CAM procedure. Walch type B2 and C glenoids, smaller preoperative joint space, higher radiographic grades of osteoarthritis, and age greater than 50 years have been found to be correlated with early failure.[35,50] Large inferior humeral head osteophytes have been associated with inferior outcomes.[34] It is postulated that the inferior humeral head osteophyte limits abduction by tensioning the axillary pouch and is capable of compressing the axillary nerve, resulting in posterior and inferior shoulder pain and weakness.[44] There is also a possible association between the size of the inferior humeral head osteophyte and compressive neuropathy of the axillary nerve. In a retrospective review of 91 shoulders by Millett and colleagues,[45] a larger humeral head osteophyte was associated with more fatty infiltration of the teres minor. However, age was also found to be associated with increased fatty infiltration. Incorporating humeral head osteoplasty and axillary nerve decompression into the standard arthroscopic management of glenohumeral arthritis may explain the difference in outcomes with the CAM procedure.

Conversely, other studies have shown that isolated arthroscopic debridement and capsular release without any other procedure are associated with only temporary pain relief and improvement in motion.[51,52] In 1 retrospective review of 33 patients who underwent arthroscopic debridement and capsular release, Skelley and colleagues[51] reported that although there was an initial improvement in pain scores and range of motion, patients returned to preoperative levels approximately 3.8 months postoperatively. Additionally, 60.6% of patients were not satisfied with the procedure, and total shoulder arthroplasty was undertaken in 42.4% of patients at an average of 8.8 months postoperatively.

In regards to microfracture, studies with short-term follow-up of patients with microfracture of glenohumeral articular defects have shown promising results, with significant improvements in pain relief and shoulder function.[22,53,54] In 1 study with a mean 10-year follow-up, Wang and colleagues[55] reported that 21.4% of patients required conversion to arthroplasty less than 10 years after the index microfracture procedure, and 33% to 42% of patients were considered to have clinical failure. However, for those patients without conversion to arthroplasty, the functional improvements were maintained between short-term and long-term follow-up. However, these studies are limited by small numbers of patients being studied. Data from Millett and colleagues[36] have also shown promising results with microfracture. In 1 study of 31 shoulders in 30 patients and mean 47-month follow-up, failure occurred in 19% of shoulders. However, in the remaining patients, there was significant improvement in functional outcome scores. Outcomes were worse with larger lesions and with bipolar lesions.

SUMMARY

Glenohumeral arthritis in the young adult is a particularly disabling condition for which optimal treatment algorithms have yet to be established. Arthroscopic joint-preserving treatments have the advantage of delaying arthroplasty in this younger population while maintaining the patient's natural anatomy and do not appear to compromise later arthroplasty. Various surgical techniques are available such that the overall procedure is tailored to the patient's individual pathology. These procedures include joint debridement, chondroplasty, microfracture, synovectomy, loose body removal, capsular releases, subacromial decompression, subcoracoid decompression, biceps tenodesis/tenotomy, humeral osteoplasty, and potential axillary nerve decompression. Short- and medium-term studies show good outcomes with low conversion to total shoulder arthroplasty and sustained improvements in functional outcome scores. Further studies are needed to establish long-term outcomes and better define the role for these procedures.

REFERENCES

1. Centers for Disease Control and Prevention (CDC). Prevalence and most common causes of disability among adults—United States, 2005. MMWR Morb Mortal Wkly Rep 2009;58:421–6.
2. Gartsman GM, Brinker MR, Khan M, et al. Self-assessment of general health status in patients with five common shoulder conditions. J Shoulder Elbow Surg 1998;7:228–37.
3. Carter MJ, Mikuls TR, Nayak S, et al. Impact of total shoulder arthroplasty on generic and shoulder-specific health-related quality of life measures: a systematic literature review and meta-analysis. J Bone Joint Surg Am 2012;94:e127.
4. Denard PJ, Wirth MA, Orfaly RM. Management of glenohumeral arthritis in the young adult. J Bone Joint Surg Am 2011;93:885–92.

5. Puzzitiello RN, Agarwalla A, Liu JN, et al. Establishing maximal medical improvement after anatomic total shoulder arthroplasty. J Shoulder Elbow Surg 2018;27:1711–20.

6. Simovitch RW, Friedman RJ, Cheung EV, et al. Rate of improvement in clinical outcomes with anatomic and reverse total shoulder arthroplasty. J Bone Joint Surg Am 2017;99:1801–11.

7. Baumgarten KM, Chang PS, Dannenbring TM, et al. Does total shoulder arthroplasty improve patients' activity levels? J Shoulder Elbow Surg 2018; 27:1987–95.

8. Boselli KJ, Ahmad CS, Levine WN. Treatment of glenohumeral arthrosis. Am J Sports Med 2010; 38:2558–72.

9. Saltzman MD, Mercer DM, Warme WJ, et al. Comparison of patients undergoing primary shoulder arthroplasty before and after age fifty. J Bone Joint Surg Am 2010;92:42–7.

10. Sperling JW, Antuna SA, Sanchez-Sotelo J, et al. Shoulder arthroplasty for arthritis after instability surgery. J Bone Joint Surg Am 2002;84:1775–81.

11. Sperling JW, Cofield RH, Rowland CM. Neer hemiarthroplasty and Neer total shoulder arthroplasty in patients fifty years old or less. Long-term results. J Bone Joint Surg Am 1998;80:464–73.

12. Roberson TA, Bentley JC, Griscom JT, et al. Outcomes of total shoulder arthroplasty in patients younger than 65 years: a systematic review. J Shoulder Elbow Surg 2017;26:1298–306.

13. Takamura KM, Chen JB, Petrigliano FA. Nonarthroplasty options for the athlete or active individual with shoulder osteoarthritis. Clin Sports Med 2018;37:517–26.

14. Denard PJ, Raiss P, Sowa B, et al. Mid- to long-term follow-up of total shoulder arthroplasty using a keeled glenoid in young adults with primary glenohumeral arthritis. J Shoulder Elbow Surg 2013;22: 894–900.

15. Schoch B, Schleck C, Cofield RH, et al. Shoulder arthroplasty in patients younger than 50 years: minimum 20-year follow-up. J Shoulder Elbow Surg 2015;24:705–10.

16. Burkhart S, Lo IKY, Brady PC, et al. Glenohumeral arthritis. In: Burkhart SS, editor. The cowboy's companion: a trail guide for the arthroscopic shoulder surgeon. Philadelphia: Wolters Kluwer; 2012. p. 410–9.

17. Millett PJ, Fritz EM, Frangiamore SJ, et al. Arthroscopic management of glenohumeral arthritis: a joint preservation approach. J Am Acad Orthop Surg 2018;26:745–52.

18. Henn RF, Ghomrawi H, Rutledge JR, et al. Preoperative patient expectations of total shoulder arthroplasty. J Bone Joint Surg Am 2011;93: 2110–5.

19. Garcia GH, Taylor SA, DePalma BJ, et al. Patient activity levels after reverse total shoulder arthroplasty:

what are patients doing? Am J Sports Med 2015;43: 2816–21.

20. Garcia GH, Liu JN, Sinatro A, et al. High satisfaction and return to sports after total shoulder arthroplasty in patients ages 55 years and younger. Am J Sports Med 2017;45:1664–9.

21. Mannava S, Horan MP, Frangiamore SJ, et al. Return to recreational sporting activities following total shoulder arthroplasty. Orthop J Sports Med 2018;6:1–7.

22. Sayegh ET, Mascarenhas R, Chalmers PN, et al. Surgical treatment options for glenohumeral arthritis in young patients: a systematic review and meta-analysis. Arthroscopy 2015;31:1156–66.

23. Elhassan B, Ozbaydar M, Diller D, et al. Soft-tissue resurfacing of the glenoid in the treatment of glenohumeral arthritis in active patients less than fifty years old. J Bone Joint Surg Am 2009;91:419–24.

24. Bhat SB, Lazarus M, Getz C, et al. Economic decision model suggests total shoulder arthroplasty is superior to hemiarthroplasty in young patients with end-stage shoulder arthritis. Clin Orthop Relat Res 2016;474:2482–92.

25. Padegimas EM, Maltenfort M, Lazarus MD, et al. Future patient demand for shoulder arthroplasty by younger patients: national projections. Clin Orthop Relat Res 2015;473:1860–7.

26. Busfield BT, Romero DM. Pain pump use after shoulder arthroscopy as a cause of glenohumeral chondrolysis. Arthroscopy 2009;25:647–52.

27. Yeh PC, Kharrazi FD. Postarthroscopic glenohumeral chondrolysis. J Am Acad Orthop Surg 2012; 20:102–12.

28. Kerr R, Resnick D, Pineda C, et al. Osteoarthritis of the glenohumeral joint: a radiologic-pathologic study. AJR Am J Roentgenol 1985;144:967–72.

29. Kircher J, Morhard M, Magosch P, et al. How much are radiological parameters related to clinical symptoms and function in osteoarthritis of the shoulder? Int Orthop 2010;34:677–81.

30. Cole BJ, Yanke A, Provencher MT. Nonarthroplasty alternatives for the treatment of glenohumeral arthritis. J Shoulder Elbow Surg 2007;16:S231–40.

31. Izquierdo R, Voloshin I, Edwards S, et al. Treatment of glenohumeral osteoarthritis. J Am Acad Orthop Surg 2010;18:375–82.

32. Chillemi C, Franceschini V. Shoulder osteoarthritis. Arthritis 2013;2013:370231.

33. Spiegl UJ, Faucett SC, Horan MP, et al. The role of arthroscopy in the management of glenohumeral osteoarthritis: a Markov decision model. Arthroscopy 2014;30:1392–9.

34. Weinstein DM, Bucchieri JS, Pollock RG, et al. Arthroscopic debridement of the shoulder for osteoarthritis. Arthroscopy 2000;16:471–6.

35. Van Thiel GS, Sheehan S, Frank RM, et al. Retrospective analysis of arthroscopic management of

glenohumeral degenerative disease. Arthroscopy 2010;26:1451–5.

36. Millett PJ, Huffard BH, Horan MP, et al. Outcomes of full-thickness articular cartilage injuries of the shoulder treated with microfracture. Arthroscopy 2009;25:856–63.

37. Warner BT, Horan MP, Raynor MB, et al. Arthroscopic management of glenohumeral osteoarthritis: prospective evaluation of factors associated with success. Presented at the Arthroscopy Association of North America Annual Meeting. Los Angeles, CA, 2015.

38. Steadman JR, Rodkey WG, Rodrigo JJ. Microfracture: surgical technique and rehabilitation to treat chondral defects. Clin Orthop Relat Res 2001; 391S:S362–9.

39. Provencher MT, Barker JU, Strauss EJ, et al. Glenohumeral arthritis in the young adult. Instr Course Lect 2011;60:137–53.

40. Mook WR, Petri M, Greenspoon JA, et al. The comprehensive arthroscopic management procedure for treatment of glenohumeral osteoarthritis. Arthrosc Tech 2015;4:e435–41.

41. Millett PJ, Horan MP, Pennock AT, et al. Comprehensive arthroscopic management (CAM) procedure: clinical results of a joint-preserving arthroscopic treatment for young, active patients with advanced shoulder osteoarthritis. Arthroscopy 2013;29:440–8.

42. Lo IK, Burkhart SS. Arthroscopic coracoplasty through the rotator cuff interval. Arthroscopy 2003;19:667–71.

43. Millett PJ, Gaskill TR. Arthroscopic trans-capsular axillary nerve decompression: indication and surgical technique. Arthroscopy 2011;27:1444–8.

44. Millett PJ, Gaskill TR. Arthroscopic management of glenohumeral arthrosis: humeral osteoplasty, capsular release, and arthroscopic axillary nerve release as a joint-preserving approach. Arthroscopy 2011;27:1296–303.

45. Millett PJ, Schoenahl JY, Allen MJ, et al. An association between the inferior humeral head osteophyte and teres minor fatty infiltration: evidence for axillary nerve entrapment in glenohumeral osteoarthritis. J Shoulder Elbow Surg 2013;22: 215–21.

46. Ogilvie-Harris DJ, Wiley AM. Arthroscopic surgery of the shoulder. A general appraisal. J Bone Joint Surg Br 1986;68:201–7.

47. Cameron BD, Galatz LM, Ramsey ML, et al. Non-prosthetic management of grade IV osteochondral lesions of the glenohumeral joint. J Shoulder Elbow Surg 2002;11:25–32.

48. Kerr BJ, McCarty EC. Outcome of arthroscopic debridement is worse for patients with glenohumeral arthritis of both sides of the joint. Clin Orthop Relat Res 2008;466:634–8.

49. Mitchell JJ, Horan MP, Greenspoon JA, et al. Survivorship and patient-reported outcomes after comprehensive arthroscopic management of glenohumeral osteoarthritis: minimum 5-year follow-up. Am J Sports Med 2016;44:3206–13.

50. Mitchell JJ, Warner BT, Horan MP, et al. Comprehensive arthroscopic management of glenohumeral osteoarthritis: preoperative factors predictive of treatment failure. Am J Sports Med 2017;45: 794–802.

51. Skelley NW, Namdari S, Chamberlain AM, et al. Arthroscopic debridement and capsular release for the treatment of shoulder osteoarthritis. Arthroscopy 2015;31:494–500.

52. Namdari S, Skelley N, Kenner JD, et al. What is the role of arthroscopic debridement for glenohumeral arthritis? A critical evaluation of the literature. Arthroscopy 2013;29:1392–8.

53. Frank RM, Van Thiel GS, Slabaugh MA, et al. Clinical outcomes after microfracture of the glenohumeral joint. Am J Sports Med 2010;38: 771–81.

54. Snow M, Funk L. Microfracture of chondral lesions of the glenohumeral joint. Int J Shoulder Surg 2008;2:72–6.

55. Wang KC, Frank RM, Cotter EJ, et al. Long-term clinical outcomes after microfracture of the glenohumeral joint: average 10-year follow-up. Am J Sports Med 2018;46:786–94.

Foot and Ankle

Pathogenesis of Posttraumatic Osteoarthritis of the Ankle

Eugene C. Nwankwo Jr, MS[a,b], Lawal A. Labaran, BS[c],
Vincent Athas, BS[b], Steve Olson, MD[a],
Samuel B. Adams, MD[a,*]

KEYWORDS

- Ankle • Arthritis • Posttraumatic • Osteoarthritis • Pilon • Fracture

---

KEY POINTS

- PTOAA is most common after a traumatic injury to the ankle joint.
- Pathogenic mechanisms of PTOAA are not fully understood.
- Metabolites, lipids, and cytokines are associated with the development of PTOAA.
- Surgical reduction is the most accepted standard of treatment of PTOAA.
- Recent literature suggests possible management of PTOAA by targeting metabolites, lipids, cytokines, and oxidative stressors.

INTRODUCTION

Osteoarthritis (OA) remains one of the most common causes of chronic joint pain in adults, affecting approximately 15% of the world's adult population.[1,2] One percent of OA diagnoses involve the ankle joint.[3,4] Posttraumatic osteoarthritis (PTOA) is the most common cause of arthritis in the ankle.[4–9] Trauma accounts for a disproportionate amount of arthritis in the ankle joint compared with other joints in the body, with estimates approaching 80%.[2,3,10,11] The most common traumatic cause of PTOA is thought to be intra-articular ankle fracture leading to cartilaginous damage and ligament instability.[4,5,9,12–15] But the exact mechanism is unknown.

The treatment of PTOA in all joints continues to pose significant challenges in the efforts to reduce symptomatic pain and reduce disability in patients diagnosed with the disease. Currently, open reduction and internal fixation (ORIF), is the standard of care for displaced intra-articular ankle fractures (Fig. 1). ORIF is performed with an emphasis on anatomic reduction of the articular surface. However, ORIF does not always prevent PTOA. One might speculate that the development of PTOA is secondary to residual displacement of the articular surfaces following ORIF. With the development and implementation of advanced imaging, we expect to see a reduction in the incidence of PTOA in response to implementation of more refined surgical reconstruction techniques aimed to restore anatomic alignment. However, studies have shown some discrepancy between PTOA development and residual displacement of intra-articular fractures; indicating that other factors may be at play.[16] Dirschl and colleagues[17] reported that, despite implementing the use of anatomic reduction on articular surfaces within the ankle joint, over 20% of lower extremity fractures resulted in the development of clinically significant degenerative changes.

---

[a] Department of Orthopedic Surgery, Duke University Medical Center, 4709 Creekstone Drive, Durham, NC 27703, USA; [b] Texas Tech University School of Medicine, Texas Tech University Health Science Center, 3601 4th Street, Lubbock, TX 79430, USA; [c] University of Illinois College of Medicine, 1200 Harrison Street, Chicago, IL 60607, USA
* Corresponding author.
E-mail address: samuel.adams@duke.edu

Orthop Clin N Am 50 (2019) 529–537
https://doi.org/10.1016/j.ocl.2019.05.008

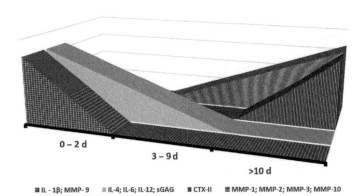

Fig. 1. Temporal composition of intra-articular mediators after ankle fracture.

0 – 2 d

3 – 9 d

>10 d

▨ IL - 1β; MMP- 9   ▨ IL-4; IL-6; IL-12; sGAG   ▨ CTX-II   ▤ MMP-1; MMP-2; MMP-3; MMP-10

Recent studies have shown that other biological factors may be of significance in the pathogenesis and therapy for PTOA of the ankle (PTOAA). Adams and colleagues[6,7] have reported increased biologic activity of inflammatory cytokines and metabolites within the synovial fluid of ankle joint after a traumatic event.[18,19] Furthermore, increased bioactivity of inflammatory cytokines was reported to have a temporal relationship on cartilage damage—with peak catabolic activity observed immediately after an ankle fracture and sustained even after bone healing.[6–8,11,20,21]

Unlike other forms of degenerative arthritis, PTOA stands out due to its specific time of onset, which means that we know when the disease process starts and therefore when to start treating it. Thus, a clear understanding of these biological events will provide improved clinical management of PTOAA. Multiple independent studies have indicated a promising link between the reduction of inflammation in the knee joint and low incidence of PTOA.[20,22,23] With the projected rise in the incidence of OA, such new evidence provides valuable insight into the complex pathogenesis of PTOA, and serves as a potential nidus in managing such a debilitating condition. In this article, we discuss recent developments that have helped to clarify some of these initial misconceptions regarding PTOAA. For the purposes of this article, ankle fractures include any intra-articular injury of the distal tibia and/or fibula (unimalleolar, bimalleolar, trimalleolar, and tibia pilon fractures).

PATHOGENESIS OF POSTTRAUMATIC ANKLE ARTHRITIS

The underlying cause of traditional OA was simply ascribed to a degenerative "wear and tear" process. A strong link has been established between obesity, metabolic syndrome, and nutrition and the incidence of OA.[24] Perhaps, these factors are most intuitive given their influence on patient weight and subsequent loading of various joints. Over the years, the multifactorial nature of traditional OA pathogenesis has become more highlighted, and stronger emphasis is now being placed on the expanding evidence that physical and biologic effects contribute to OA. However, PTOAA is different from traditional wear and tear arthritis as it starts with a substantial traumatic event. Here we will focus on the physical and physiologic aspects of the development of PTOAA.

Physical Influences in Posttraumatic Ankle Arthritis
Fracture energy and fracture reduction as contributors to posttraumatic ankle arthritis
The damage sustained at the time of injury can be objectively assessed although physical manifestations of the fracture severity: the amount of energy involved in fracturing a bone (ie, the fracture energy) and the amount of articular surface involvement. It has been demonstrated in fractures of the tibial plafond that these fracture severity metrics significantly correlate with PTOAA incidence.[25–27] This provides a possible explanation for differences found in the rates of PTOA development in tibial pilon and plateau fractures; that is, greater energy is absorbed in creating tibial pilon fractures compared with plateau fractures.

The mechanisms of these injuries are often similar. However tibial pilon fractures have a higher risk of PTOA development as opposed to fractures of the tibial plateau.[28,29] Comparisons of the joint size, articular surface, and morphology may account for the differences in

PTOA incidence between these fractures. The tibial plateau has a much larger articulating surface (~ 1200 mm^2) compared with the tibial pilon (~ 600 mm^2).[30,31] Thus, the tibio-talar joint may transmit higher energy per unit area to the intra-articular tissues (cartilage and synovium) than the tibio-femoral joint. This higher energy density results in more profound chondrocyte damage and death in the pilon in comparison with the plateau.[32]

Operative treatment has been the established standard of care for fractures. Nonetheless, the success of operative treatment depends on the occurrence of osteoarthritis postoperatively, type of fracture, and quality of fracture reduction. In a recent 7-year retrospective study of 137 fractures, Rubio-Suarez and colleagues[33] showed that certain variables (infection, suboptimal anatomic reduction) were related to a higher prevalence of nonunion and posttraumatic ankle osteoarthritis. Given that quality of fracture reduction can be modified, efforts should be made to restore articular congruence to improve the outcome.

Biomechanical differences of the ankle that influence posttraumatic ankle arthritis
The anatomy and structural differences observed in ankle fractures are well known. Although OA has been well studied in the knee, the variable rate of development of PTOA among joints could differ in their metabolism, articular surface thickness, and biomechanical properties.[14,34] Chondrocytes in human ankle cadavers joints have increased proteoglycan content and rates of collagen turnover in comparison with knee chondrocytes.[35] The increased turnover may allow ankle chondrocytes to adapt and remodel to traditional atraumatic wear and tear arthritis compared with knee chondrocytes. Aurich and colleagues[36] demonstrated that the sequence of OA disease progression includes a paradoxical increase in collagen synthesis in the damaged ankle and collagen degradation in the knee. Ankle chondrocytes have also been found to be more resistant to catabolic effects of interleukin-1β (IL-1β) or fibronectin than those in the knee.[37] This has been attributed to the influence of BMP-7.[38] Lastly, ankle cartilage has been found to be much stiffer,[39] yet thinner (1–1.45 mm) than knee cartilage (3–6 mm).[40] These congruent joints and thinner cartilages have a lower incidence of osteoarthritis.[39] These qualities may afford ankle cartilage greater resistance to compressive loads.

Physiologic Contributors to Posttraumatic Ankle Arthritis and the Inflammatory Microenvironment
There is an increasing body of literature describing the physiologic contribution to PTOAA. Recent studies suggest that the microenvironment of the osteoarthritic joint involves significant amplification of the inflammatory state within the cartilage, subchondral bone, and synovium.[6,7,11,21,41] The literature suggests evidence that a proinflammatory and oxidative microenvironment exists within the synovial fluid after ankle fractures.[6–8,19,42,43] In a comparison of 21 patients who sustained intra-articular ankle fractures, Adams and colleagues[6,8] measured cytokines and matrix metalloproteinases (MMPs) including granulocyte-macrophage colony-stimulating factor (GM-CSF), IL-10, IL-1β, IL-6, IL-8, tumor necrosis factor alpha (TNF-α), MMP-1, MMP-2, MMP-3, MMP-9, and MMP-10. As indicated in **Fig. 2**, incidence of cytokines was found to increase acutely after ankle fracture. Some remained elevated for days to months after injury, providing evidence of a persistent inflammatory environment in synovial fluid after injury. Another study suggested marked differences in lipid levels among the joint metabolome.[7,19]

More recently, Martin and his colleagues came forward with evidence that various signals and enzymes may play crucial roles in the characteristic inflammation, mitochondrial loss, and chondrocyte death observed as a response to OA and joint trauma.[43] Overall, such a body of evidence lends more credence to the increased understanding about the role of inflammation and biological pathways in PTOAA. Moreover, these pathways may serve as potential targets for nonsurgical management.

Metabolites and Lipids
Metabolomics is the quantitative analysis of large amounts of metabolites and end-products within an environment. This process is accomplished via mass spectrometry, chromatography, nuclear magnetic resonance, and other methods. Levels of metabolites can often serve to better understand a biological system's response to genotypic, phenotypic, and environmental changes, such as those that might occur in PTOA. Given their anatomic proximity in the joint, cartilage and synovium share close communication. Indeed, the synovial fluid acts as a repository for metabolic by-products of chondrocyte and synoviocyte metabolism. Therefore, a sample of the synovial fluid could indicate the overall health of the intra-articular

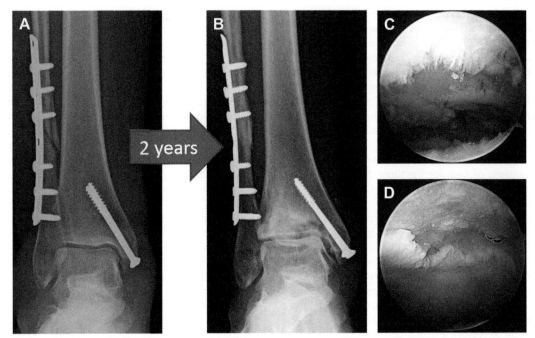

Fig. 2. (A) Anteroposterior (AP) radiograph of an intra-articular ankle fracture with anatomic reduction and fixation. (B) AP radiograph of the same ankle 2 years later demonstrating the development of arthritis throughout the ankle. (C, D) Arthroscopic images of the same ankle at 2 years, which demonstrate diffuse cartilage damage.

environment at any given time. Compared with the genome or proteome, the metabolome reflects *acute*, or *real-time*, changes occurring in biological systems. This makes the synovial metabolic profile an ideal technique to identify intra-articular environmental changes that occur after traumatic injury to the ankle joint.[19,44]

Intra-articular structures are lubricated by the presence of lipids within the synovial fluid.[45] These lipids have been associated with OA.[45,46] Specific lipids have been correlated to damage of various structures within the joint. Intra-articular fat pads yield increased triglycerides,[46] whereas damage to other structures yields a profile with reduced levels of triglycerides and elevated phospholipids.[47] A recent study characterized the metabolic profile of 19 patients after intra-articular ankle fracture with emphasis on changes in lipid levels. Baseline levels of free fatty acids [FAs], sphingomyelins, and lysolipids were found to be significantly elevated in fractured ankles. There were marked differences in long chain FA, polyunsaturated FA, and monohydroxy levels in fractured ankles at baseline compared with 6 months postsurgery.[19] Further characterization of synovial profiles indicated significant correlations between lipid metabolites and secreted cytokines based on the severity of intra-articular fractures. The authors defined the severity of ankle fractures

as follows: patients with isolated fibula or medial malleolus fracture, or fibula fracture with deltoid and/or syndesmotic ligament tear, were classified as stage 1; any bimalleolar fracture (fibula plus medial malleolus fractures) was classified as stage 2; stage 3 was reserved for trimalleolar fractures or any fracture involving the posterior malleolus. Stages 2 and 3 ankle fractures were associated with higher levels of specific lipids (medium chain FAs, lysolipids, and inositol metabolites) compared with stage 1 fractures. Lastly, soft tissue injuries, in concurrence with intra-articular ankle fractures, were associated with high levels of sphingolipid metabolites, lysolipids, dicarboxylic FAs, and ketones.[19]

Inflammatory Cytokines as Biomarkers in Posttraumatic Ankle Arthritis

Intra-articular inflammation plays a vital role in the development and progression of PTOAA. Adams and colleagues[8] recently shed some light on the acute and chronic behavior of certain proinflammatory cytokines in intra-articular inflammation. Earlier studies suggested acute increases in cytokines and MMPs, including GM-CSF, IL-10, IL-1β, IL-6, IL-8, TNF-α, MMP-1, MMP-2, MMP-3, MMP-9, and MMP-10.[6,8] These factors were significantly elevated, with peaks within 8 to 40 days after ankle fracture. Some factors remained elevated well beyond the acute window. IL-6, IL-8, and MMP-1, 2, and 3, were found to remain at elevated levels even after complete healing of the fracture. Particularly, IL-6, IL-8, and MMP-2 showed the highest quantities at 6 months following intra-articular injury.[8,11] MMP-1, MMP-3, MMP-9, and MMP-10 exhibited a less aggressive increase at the 6-month mark than other studied cytokines.[8] These observations suggest a marked presence of highly inflammatory molecules that persist in previously fractured yet healed ankles. Historically, IL-6 and IL-8 have been classified as anti- and proinflammatory cytokines,[48,49] these molecules are well-documented as markers of joint destruction in other joints and likely play a major role in the development of ankle PTOA.[48,50]

Similar to knees following an anterior cruciate ligament injury, IL-1β and TNF-α are present at equivalent levels after ankle fractures as they are at baseline.[51] This serves as evidence that cytokine levels return to baseline after knee or ankle injuries. Despite a quick return to normal, it is very possible that the deleterious effects of the subsequently activated signaling pathways may have more prolonged consequences. Given this idea, Furman and colleagues[42] provided evidence that anti-IL-1β therapy attenuates arthritis by reducing disease severity when given acutely after intra-articular fracture in mice.

NOVEL IDEAS ON THE CLINICAL MANAGEMENT OF POSTTRAUMATIC ANKLE ARTHRITIS

Traditionally accepted treatment of articular fractures in ankles involves restoration of the articular surface, correction of axial and rotational alignment of the injured limb, and surgical fixation.[52] Regardless of the quality of articular reduction, there remains variable susceptibility to the development of PTOA after intra-articular fractures.[52] Certainly, 80% of the surgically treated ankle fractures cannot be malreduced at the time of ORIF. Moreover, there is seemingly a finite amount of improvement that we, as surgeons, can accomplish on our reduction and fixation techniques. For example, McKinley and colleagues[53] reported no change in the percent of ideal clinical outcomes over the past 40+ years. Therefore, the next logical step would be to counteract the processes discussed above that are known to be present at the time of injury.

Inhibiting Oxidative Stressors
Many studies have proposed reactive oxygen species (ROS) as an important cause of OA

development. High impact load and elevated levels of ROS in injured chondrocytes are shown to induce oxidative stress, which leads to oxidization and disruption of cell homeostasis.[54–60] Numerous studies have demonstrated that MMPs play a vital role in joint cartilage disruption. Among the most important enzymes are MMP-3 and MMP-13 (which are elevated after ankle fracture). Damage induced by MMPs leads to pathologic production of excess ROS and superoxide (a secondary metabolite). These products subsequently activate transcription factors, such as nuclear factor kappa-light-chain-enhancer of activated B cells (NF-κB). Following NF-κB activation, various proinflammatory cytokines and chemokines are ultimately expressed downstream of the signaling pathway.[61,62]

Antioxidants have recently emerged as potential agents in OA but not PTOA management. Recently, Chen and colleagues[63] showed that antioxidants such as flavonoids have the capability to relieve OA in rats through the attenuation of ROS (superoxide anion, hydroxyl radical, and peroxynitrite) generation. Further, they observed suppressed levels of IL-1β-induced accumulation of NO, MMP-3, and MMP-13 by the flavonoid compound. Their studies also showed a reversal of mitochondrial dysfunction associated with chondrocyte damage and OA. Other studies seem to support the findings by Chen and colleagues that IL-1β-induced inflammatory response of OA can be subdued. These findings provide a viable therapeutic avenue for the potential treatment of PTOAA.

Cytokine Inhibition as a Viable Means of Therapy
The association between inflammasomes, cytokines, and OA pathogenesis remainstopic of discussion for many years. There is a growing body of literature indicating that higher-than-normal synthesis of interleukins plays a significant role in the progression of PTOA. To understand this correlation with joint degeneration, Olson and colleagues[64] performed studies, the results of which suggest that attenuation of the IL-1β response with an IL-1β receptor antagonist limits inflammatory response after injury, and thus may play a role in reducing the incidence of PTOA after trauma to the joint. Data from the aforementioned studies also indicated that a one-time dose of intra-articular anakinra (IL-1Ra) leads to significantly reduced cartilage degeneration in the fractured knee compared with nontreated groups.[42]

Kimmerling and colleagues[65] further elucidated on the impact of temporal administration of intra-articular cytokine inhibitors as a promising pathway for prevention or intervention against OA degeneration. Studies were conducted by administering soluble IL-1Ra and TNF receptor II inhibitors with and without an encapsulating, thermo-responsive drug depot (elastin-like polypeptide). Drug depots have been linked to a 25-fold improvement in intra-articular drug half-life. Depot-assisted delivery of cytokine inhibition showed a significant reduction in arthritic changes after 8 weeks.[23] The observation that postinjury administration of intra-articular IL-1Ra prevented arthritic changes ushers in strong evidence of a potential biologic intervention, in concert with surgical intervention, as a potential therapy for posttraumatic ankle OA.

The Promise of Tissue Engineering

In recent years, there has been a steep rise in the use of stem cell tissue engineering for the treatment of articular damage.[66] Transplantation of bone marrow-derived mesenchymal stem cells[67] and adipose-derived mesenchymal stem cells[68] has been at the forefront of efforts to broaden the arsenal against diseases associated with damaged cartilage. Induction of cell homing without transplantation has also led to notable success in regard to cartilage repair.[69] Studies have been able to identify stem/progenitor cells, chondrogenic progenitor cells (CPCs), in articular cartilage, and repair tissue in end-stage OA.[70–72] These cells are now known to respond to various cytokines and chemokines, allowing migration toward damaged cartilage tissues and subsequent repair of cartilage defects.[72–74] Although there remains poor evidence that CPCs regenerate articular cartilage, these cells carry a promise to bring stem cell and tissue engineering to the frontline in the quest to reduce the progression of PTOA in knees and ankles.

Despite advances in tissue engineering and biotechnology, these methods fall short in their ability to fully restore human articular cartilage to full vitality. Lower cell yields, phenotypic differences, and variance in chondrogenic activity remain a hindrance in tissue engineering therapy.[75] Yu and colleagues showed significant improvements in this strategy of cartilage by enhancing the recruitment of migratory progenitor cells to the interpenetrating polymer network using recombinant human SDF-1a, followed by treatments to initiate chondrogenic differentiation. This was done with the assistance of a stem cell scaffold with very similar characteristics to native cartilage and, as such, possesses mechanical properties within the physiologic range of functional native cartilage. Further improvements and optimization of this method could serve as a foundation for a less-invasive procedure to repair damaged cartilage in PTOA.

SUMMARY

The objective of this review was to further clarify the current understanding of PTOAA pathogenesis and management. We aimed to provide a comprehensive discussion of the biological factors influencing the development and advancement of PTOAA. This review has demonstrated that there are a variety of factors that influence the development and severity of PTOAA. Some of the most notable of these were the role of fracture energy distribution, the biomechanics of the ankle joint, proinflammatory cytokines, and metabolites.

The pathogenesis of PTOAA remains poorly understood. Treppo and colleagues[39] established that joint congruence and cartilage thickness may confer greater protection against osteoarthritis as these factors may alter the load and compression experienced by the ankle joint. They reported that chondrocytes in the ankle are more resistant to catabolism by IL-1β and other proinflammatory cytokines. A more recent study by Anderson and colleagues[27] further suggested that a smaller articular surface area in the tibial pilon may facilitate a higher fracture energy density in the distal tibia and ankle as opposed to the proximal tibia and tibio-femoral joint.[25,26] Such increased energy leads to more prominent chondrocyte damage and death in the pilon.[32] These narratives may provide a strong explanation for the much higher incidence of PTOAA than OA at other joints. At the molecular level, the assessment of the synovial fluid components by Adams and colleagues[11,21] indicates an acute increase in key cytokines and MMPs in the ankle joint after intra-articular ankle fractures.[19] Sustained levels of these cytokines and metabolites in the days and months after injury may further facilitate development and severe progression of PTOAA. In fact, these studies showed a correlation between higher levels of lipid metabolites (medium chain FAs, lysolipids, and inositol) to more severe stages of an ankle injury.

Various mechanisms involved in the development and progression of PTOAA have been proposed as potential markers and targets for therapy. Inhibition of inflammatory cytokines with unique activity in the ankle may serve as a viable means of disease treatment and modification. Olson and colleagues[64] elucidated that the attenuation of IL-1β and TNF-α response with receptor antagonists reduces inflammation and cartilage degeneration within the ankle joint after a traumatic event.[23] Most recently, rising interest in stem cell bioengineering has led to studies on cell lines that may facilitate tissue repair through enhanced recruitment and differentiation of chondrocytes in OA-afflicted ankle joints.[69,71–73] These observations offer strong evidence of a potential biologic intervention to reverse the progression of OA. In concert with surgical intervention as a potential therapy, pharmacologic agents may serve to augment and improve the incidence and severity of posttraumatic ankle OA.

REFERENCES

1. Johnson VL, Hunter DJ. The epidemiology of osteoarthritis. Best Pract Res Clin Rheumatol 2014. https://doi.org/10.1016/j.berh.2014.01.004.

2. Felson DT. An update on the pathogenesis and epidemiology of osteoarthritis. Radiol Clin North Am 2004. https://doi.org/10.1016/S0033-8389(03)00161-1.

3. Peyron JG. Osteoarthritis. The epidemiologic viewpoint. Clin Orthop Relat Res 1986;(213):13–9.

4. Weatherall JM, Mroczek K, McLaurin T, et al. Posttraumatic ankle arthritis. Bull Hosp Jt Dis (2013) 2013;71(1):104–12.

5. Valderrabano V, Horisberger M, Russell I, et al. Etiology of ankle osteoarthritis. Clin Orthop Relat Res 2009. https://doi.org/10.1007/s11999-008-0543-6.

6. Adams SB, Setton LA, Bell RD, et al. Inflammatory cytokines and matrix metalloproteinases in the synovial fluid after intra-articular ankle fracture. Foot Ankle Int 2015. https://doi.org/10.1177/1071100715611176.

7. Adams SB, Nettles DL, Jones LC, et al. Inflammatory cytokines and cellular metabolites as synovial fluid biomarkers of posttraumatic ankle arthritis. Foot Ankle Int 2014. https://doi.org/10.1177/1071100714550652.

8. Adams SB, Leimer EM, Setton LA, et al. Inflammatory microenvironment persists after bone healing in intra-articular ankle fractures. Foot Ankle Int 2017. https://doi.org/10.1177/1071100717690427.

9. Furman BD, Olson SA, Guilak F. The development of posttraumatic arthritis after articular fracture. J Orthop Trauma 2006. https://doi.org/10.1097/01.bot.0000211160.05864.14.

10. Brown TD, Johnston RC, Saltzman CL, et al. Posttraumatic osteoarthritis: a first estimate of incidence, prevalence, and burden of disease. J Orthop Trauma 2006. https://doi.org/10.1097/01.bot.0000246468.80635.ef.

11. Adams SB, Reilly RM, Huebner JL, et al. Time-dependent effects on synovial fluid composition during the acute phase of human intra-articular ankle fracture. Foot Ankle Int 2017. https://doi.org/10.1177/1071100717728234.

12. Horisberger M, Valderrabano V, Hintermann B. Posttraumatic ankle osteoarthritis after ankle-related fractures. J Orthop Trauma 2009. https://doi.org/10.1097/BOT.0b013e31818915d9.

13. Valderrabano V, Hintermann B, Horisberger M, et al. Ligamentous posttraumatic ankle osteoarthritis. Am J Sports Med 2006. https://doi.org/10.1177/0363546505281813.

14. Saltzman CL, Salamon ML, Blanchard GM, et al. Epidemiology of ankle arthritis: report of a consecutive series of 639 patients from a tertiary orthopaedic center. Iowa Orthop J 2005;25:44–6.

15. Wikstrom EA, Hubbard-Turner T, McKeon PO. Understanding and treating lateral ankle sprains and their consequences: a constraints-based approach. Sports Med 2013. https://doi.org/10.1007/s40279-013-0043-z.

16. Giannoudis PV, Tzioupis C, Papathanassopoulos A, et al. Articular step-off and risk of post-traumatic osteoarthritis. Evidence today. Injury 2010. https://doi.org/10.1016/j.injury.2010.08.003.

17. Dirschl DR, Marsh JL, Buckwalter JA, et al. Articular fractures. J Am Acad Orthop Surg 2004. https://doi.org/10.5435/00124635-200411000-00006.

18. Furman BD, Kimmerling KA, Zura RD, et al. Brief report: articular ankle fracture results in increased synovitis, synovial macrophage infiltration, and synovial fluid concentrations of inflammatory cytokines and chemokines. Arthritis Rheumatol 2015. https://doi.org/10.1002/art.39064.

19. Leimer EM, Pappan KL, Nettles DL, et al. Lipid profile of human synovial fluid following intra-articular ankle fracture. J Orthop Res 2017. https://doi.org/10.1002/jor.23217.

20. Allen KD, Adams SB, Mata BA, et al. Gait and behavior in an IL1β-mediated model of rat knee arthritis and effects of an IL1 antagonist. J Orthop Res 2011. https://doi.org/10.1002/jor.21309.

21. Adams SB, Setton LA, Kensicki E, et al. Global metabolic profiling of human osteoarthritic synovium. Osteoarthr Cartil 2012. https://doi.org/10.1016/j.joca.2011.10.010.

22. Ward BD, Furman BD, Huebner JL, et al. Absence of posttraumatic arthritis following intraarticular fracture in the MRL/MpJ mouse. Arthritis Rheum 2008. https://doi.org/10.1002/art.23288.

23. Lewis JS, Furman BD, Zeitler E, et al. Genetic and cellular evidence of decreased inflammation associated with reduced incidence of posttraumatic

arthritis in MRL/MpJ mice. Arthritis Rheum 2013. https://doi.org/10.1002/art.37796.

24. Bortoluzzi A, Furini F, Scirè CA. Osteoarthritis and its management-epidemiology, nutritional aspects and environmental factors. Autoimmun Rev 2018. https://doi.org/10.1016/j.autrev.2018.06.002.

25. Thomas TP, Anderson DD, Mosqueda TV, et al. Objective CT-based metrics of articular fracture severity to assess risk for posttraumatic osteoarthritis. J Orthop Trauma 2010. https://doi.org/10.1097/BOT.0b013e3181d7a0aa.

26. Thomas TP, Anderson DD, Marsh JL, et al. A method for the estimation of normative bone surface area to aid in objective CT-based fracture severity assessment. Iowa Orthop J 2008.

27. Anderson DD, Mosqueda T, Thomas T, et al. Quantifying tibial plafond fracture severity: absorbed energy and fragment displacement agree with clinical rank ordering. J Orthop Res 2008. https://doi.org/10.1002/jor.20550.

28. Honkonen SE. Degenerative arthritis after tibial plateau fractures. J Orthop Trauma 1995. https://doi.org/10.1097/00005131-199509040-00001.

29. Volpin G, Dowd GS, Stein H, et al. Degenerative arthritis after intra-articular fractures of the knee. Long-term results. J Bone Joint Surg Br 1990; 72(4):634–8.

30. Fukubayashi T, Kurosawa H. the contact area and pressure distribution pattern of the knee: a study of normal and osteoarthrotic knee joints. Acta Orthop 1980. https://doi.org/10.3109/17453678008990887.

31. Li W, Anderson DD, Goldsworthy JK, et al. Patient-specific finite element analysis of chronic contact stress exposure after intraarticular fracture of the tibial plafond. J Orthop Res 2008. https://doi.org/10.1002/jor.20642.

32. Dibbern K, Kempton LB, Higgins TF, et al. Fractures of the tibial plateau involve similar energies as the tibial pilon but greater articular surface involvement. J Orthop Res 2017. https://doi.org/10.1002/jor.23359.

33. Rubio-Suarez J, Carbonell-Escobar R, Rodriguez-Merchan EC, et al. Fractures of the tibial pilon treated by open reduction and internal fixation (locking compression plate-less invasive stabilising system): complications and sequelae. Int J Care Inj 2018;49(2):S60–4.

34. Delco ML, Kennedy JG, Bonassar LJ, et al. Post-traumatic osteoarthritis of the ankle: a distinct clinical entity requiring new research approaches. J Orthop Res 2017. https://doi.org/10.1002/jor.23462.

35. Huch K. Knee and ankle: human joints with different susceptibility to osteoarthritis reveal different cartilage cellularity and matrix synthesis in vitro. Arch Orthop Trauma Surg 2001. https://doi.org/10.1007/s004020000225.

36. Aurich M, Squires GR, Reiner A, et al. Differential matrix degradation and turnover in early cartilage lesions of human knee and ankle joints. Arthritis Rheum 2005. https://doi.org/10.1002/art.20740.

37. Kang Y, Koepp H, Cole AA, et al. Cultured human ankle and knee cartilage differ in susceptibility to damage mediated by fibronectin fragments. J Orthop Res 1998. https://doi.org/10.1002/jor.1100160505.

38. Hendren L, Beeson P. A review of the differences between normal and osteoarthritis articular cartilage in human knee and ankle joints. Foot 2009. https://doi.org/10.1016/j.foot.2009.03.003.

39. Treppo S, Koepp H, Quan EC, et al. Comparison of biomechanical and biochemical properties of cartilage from human knee and ankle pairs. J Orthop Res 2000. https://doi.org/10.1002/jor.1100180510.

40. Athanasiou KA, Niederauer GG, Schenck RC. Biomechanical topography of human ankle cartilage. Ann Biomed Eng 1995. https://doi.org/10.1007/BF02584467.

41. Sun ARJ, Friis T, Sekar S, et al. Is synovial macrophage activation the inflammatory link between obesity and osteoarthritis? Curr Rheumatol Rep 2016. https://doi.org/10.1007/s11926-016-0605-9.

42. Furman BD, Mangiapani DS, Zeitler E, et al. Targeting pro-inflammatory cytokines following joint injury: acute intra-articular inhibition of interleukin-1 following knee injury prevents post-traumatic arthritis. Arthritis Res Ther 2014. https://doi.org/10.1186/ar4591.

43. Coleman M, Brouillette M, Andresen N, et al. Differential effects of superoxide dismutase mimetics after mechanical overload of articular cartilage. Antioxidants 2017. https://doi.org/10.3390/antiox6040098.

44. Adams SB, Setton LA, Nettles DL. The role of metabolomics in osteoarthritis research. J Am Acad Orthop Surg 2013. https://doi.org/10.5435/JAAOS-21-01-63.

45. Kosinska MK, Liebisch G, Lochnit G, et al. A lipidomic study of phospholipid classes and species in human synovial fluid. Arthritis Rheum 2013. https://doi.org/10.1002/art.38053.

46. Rabinowitz JL, Gregg JR, Nixon JE. Lipid composition of the tissues of human knee joints. II. Synovial fluid in trauma. Clin Orthop Relat Res 1984.

47. Reginato AJ, Schumacher HR, Allan DA, et al. Acute monoarthritis associated with lipid liquid crystals. Ann Rheum Dis 1985. https://doi.org/10.1136/ard.44.8.537.

48. Wojdasiewicz P, Poniatowski ŁA, Szukiewicz D. The role of inflammatory and anti-inflammatory cytokines in the pathogenesis of osteoarthritis. Mediators Inflamm 2014. https://doi.org/10.1155/2014/561459.

49. Jawa RS, Anillo S, Huntoon K, et al. Interleukin-6 in surgery, trauma, and critical care. Part II. Clinical implications. J Intensive Care Med 2011. https://doi.org/10.1177/0885066610395679.

50. Elford PR, Cooper PH. Induction of neutrophil-mediated cartilage degradation by interleukin-8. Arthritis Rheum 1991. https://doi.org/10.1002/art.1780340310.

51. Lieberthal J, Sambamurthy N, Scanzello CR. Inflammation in joint injury and post-traumatic osteoarthritis. Osteoarthr Cartil 2015. https://doi.org/10.1016/j.joca.2015.08.015.

52. Schatzker J, Tile M, Axelrod T, et al. The rationale of operative fracture care. 3rd edition. Heidelberg (Berlin): Springer-Verlag; 2005. https://doi.org/10.1007/3-540-27708-0.

53. McKinley TO, Borrelli J, D'Lima DD, et al. Basic science of intra-articular fractures and posttraumatic osteoarthritis. J Orthop Trauma 2010. https://doi.org/10.1097/BOT.0b013e3181ed298d.

54. Henrotin YE, Bruckner P, Pujol JPL. The role of reactive oxygen species in homeostasis and degradation of cartilage. Osteoarthr Cartil 2003. https://doi.org/10.1016/S1063-4584(03)00150-X.

55. Greenwald RA, Moy WW. Effect of oxygen-derived free radicals on hyaluronic acid. Arthritis Rheum 1980. https://doi.org/10.1002/art.1780230408.

56. Martin J a, Brown T, Heiner A, et al. Post-traumatic osteoarthritis: the role of accelerated chondrocyte senescence. Biorheology 2004. https://doi.org/10.1016/j.bbadis.2006.01.005.

57. DiMicco MA, Patwari P, Siparsky PN, et al. Mechanisms and kinetics of glycosaminoglycan release following in vitro cartilage injury. Arthritis Rheum 2004. https://doi.org/10.1002/art.20101.

58. Lee JH, Fitzgerald JB, DiMicco MA, et al. Mechanical injury of cartilage explants causes specific time-dependent changes in chondrocyte gene expression. Arthritis Rheum 2005. https://doi.org/10.1002/art.21215.

59. Torzilli PA, Grigiene R, Borrelli J, et al. Effect of impact load on articular cartilage: cell metabolism and viability, and matrix water content. J Biomech Eng 1999. https://doi.org/10.1115/1.2835070.

60. Stolberg-Stolberg JA, Furman BD, William Garrigues N, et al. Effects of cartilage impact with and without fracture on chondrocyte viability and the release of inflammatory markers. J Orthop Res 2013. https://doi.org/10.1002/jor.22348.

61. Chung HY, Cesari M, Anton S, et al. Molecular inflammation: underpinnings of aging and age-related diseases. Ageing Res Rev 2009. https://doi.org/10.1016/j.arr.2008.07.002.

62. Kienhofer J, Haussler DJF, Ruckelshausen F, et al. Association of mitochondrial antioxidant enzymes with mitochondrial DNA as integral nucleoid constituents. FASEB J 2009. https://doi.org/10.1096/fj.08-113571.

63. Qiu L, Luo Y, Chen X. Quercetin attenuates mitochondrial dysfunction and biogenesis via upregulated AMPK/SIRT1 signaling pathway in OA rats. Biomed Pharmacother 2018. https://doi.org/10.1016/j.biopha.2018.05.003.

64. Olson SA, Furman BD, Kraus VB, et al. Therapeutic opportunities to prevent post-traumatic arthritis: lessons from the natural history of arthritis after articular fracture. J Orthop Res 2015. https://doi.org/10.1002/jor.22940.

65. Kimmerling KA, Furman BD, Mangiapani DS, et al. Sustained intra-articular delivery of IL-1Ra from a thermally-responsive elastin-like polypeptide as a therapy for post-traumatic arthritis. Eur Cell Mater 2015. https://doi.org/10.22203/eCM.v029a10.

66. Tuan RS. Stemming cartilage degeneration: adult mesenchymal stem cells as a cell source for articular cartilage tissue engineering. Arthritis Rheum 2006. https://doi.org/10.1002/art.22148.

67. Pittenger MF, Mackay AM, Beck SC, et al. Multilineage potential of adult human mesenchymal stem cells. Science 1999. https://doi.org/10.1126/science.284.5411.143.

68. Erickson IE, Kestle SR, Zellars KH, et al. High mesenchymal stem cell seeding densities in hyaluronic acid hydrogels produce engineered cartilage with native tissue properties. Acta Biomater 2012. https://doi.org/10.1016/j.actbio.2012.04.033.

69. Lee CH, Cook JL, Mendelson A, et al. Regeneration of the articular surface of the rabbit synovial joint by cell homing: a proof of concept study. Lancet 2010. https://doi.org/10.1016/S0140-6736(10)60668-X.

70. Dowthwaite GP. The surface of articular cartilage contains a progenitor cell population. J Cell Sci 2004. https://doi.org/10.1242/jcs.00912.

71. Alsalameh S, Amin R, Gemba T, et al. Identification of mesenchymal progenitor cells in normal and osteoarthritic human articular cartilage. Arthritis Rheum 2004. https://doi.org/10.1002/art.20269.

72. Koelling S, Kruegel J, Irmer M, et al. Migratory chondrogenic progenitor cells from repair tissue during the later stages of human osteoarthritis. Cell Stem Cell 2009. https://doi.org/10.1016/j.stem.2009.01.015.

73. Seol D, McCabe DJ, Choe H, et al. Chondrogenic progenitor cells respond to cartilage injury. Arthritis Rheum 2012. https://doi.org/10.1002/art.34613.

74. Seol D, Yu Y, Choe H, et al. Effect of short-term enzymatic treatment on cell migration and cartilage regeneration: in vitro organ culture of bovine articular cartilage. Tissue Eng Part A 2014. https://doi.org/10.1089/ten.TEA.2013.0444.

75. Yu Y, Brouillette MJ, Seol D, et al. Use of recombinant human stromal cell-derived factor 1α-loaded fibrin/hyaluronic acid hydrogel networks to achieve functional repair of full-thickness bovine articular cartilage via homing of chondrogenic progenitor cells. Arthritis Rheumatol 2015. https://doi.org/10.1002/art.39049.

Outcomes Following Total Ankle Arthroplasty
A Review of the Registry Data and Current Literature

Luckshmana Jeyaseelan, MBBS, BSc, FRCS(Tr&Orth),
Sam Si-Hyeong Park, MD, MASc, FRCSC,
Husam Al-Rumaih, MD, MPH,
Andrea Veljkovic, MD, MPH, FRCSC,
Murray J. Penner, MD, FRCSC, Kevin J. Wing, MD, FRCSC,
Alistair Younger, MB ChB, MSc, ChM, FRCSC*

KEYWORDS

- Total ankle arthroplasty • Ankle replacement • Outcomes • Prosthesis survivorship

KEY POINTS

- End-stage ankle arthritis has a significant effect on function and quality of life.
- Total ankle arthroplasty continues to emerge as a safe and effective treatment of ankle arthritis.
- With encouraging outcomes and improved implant longevity, there has been a significant improvement on the results of the first-generation implants.

INTRODUCTION

Osteoarthritis of the ankle is a major cause of disability, with an impact on quality of life similar to end-stage heart failure[1] and hip arthritis.[2] Its incidence has been estimated to be 47.7/100,000, affecting approximately 1% of the world population.[2–4] Most cases are caused by trauma and osteoarthritis, with other causes including inflammatory arthritis. The incidence of ankle sprains and fractures is increasing, with arthritis typically setting in within 2 to 22 years of injury.[5–7] Consequently, an increasing number of young adults still in their working lives are developing ankle arthritis.

The two main surgical treatments that are available to those with end-stage ankle arthritis are ankle arthrodesis and total ankle replacement. Debridement, distraction arthroplasty, and osteotomies may be of benefit, but in a limited number of select patients.

Ankle arthrodesis has, for many years, been the gold standard. However, it is well documented that tibiotalar fusions leads to deficits in function and may cause or exacerbate adjacent joint arthritis, particularly in the subtalar joint.[8,9] Ankle arthroplasty preserves motion at the ankle joint, while still achieving the primary goal of pain relief. However, the results from the first generations of total ankle replacement were disappointing because of poor clinical results and high rates of aseptic loosening.[10–13] The first-generation prostheses were nonmodular with all-polyethylene tibial components and solid metallic talar components using bone cement for the bone prosthesis interface. Current three-component mobile-bearing implants have much improved early to mid-term results,

---

Disclosures: See last page of article.
Department of Orthopaedics, University of British Columbia, Footbridge Centre for Integrated Orthopaedic Care, 221 - 181 Keefer Place, Vancouver, British Columbia V6B 6C1, Canada
* Corresponding author.
E-mail address: alastair.stephen.younger@gmail.com

Orthop Clin N Am 50 (2019) 539–548
https://doi.org/10.1016/j.ocl.2019.06.004

resulting in ankle arthroplasty being an effective option in certain patient populations.[14,15]

This article reviews the most current literature, including latest registry data, on the outcomes of the currently used total ankle replacement prostheses.

METHODS

Data from different international total ankle replacement joint registries were first collected and reviewed. These included the Swedish, Norwegian, New Zealand, Australian, and United Kingdom joint registries (Table 1). The latest annual reports were accessed and data analyzed looking at overall numbers and outcomes, and the most recent year data available.

PubMed, MEDLINE, and Google Scholar searches were then performed to identify previous meta-analyses, systematic reviews, and individual studies on specific prostheses. MeSH terms used in the searches included "ankle," "replacement," and "arthroplasty." Results were filtered to identify meta-analyses and systematic reviews as described. Literature on specific prostheses was limited to publications within the last 10 years. Other inclusion criteria were English language publications, publications with full text, and publications that specifically looked at outcomes of total ankle replacement only.

INTERNATIONAL REGISTRY DATA
The Swedish Ankle Registry
The latest data from the Swedish registry were published in The Swedish Ankle Registry Annual Report 2017.[16] In 2017, 66 primary replacements were performed, an increase of 14 from 2016. Osteoarthritis was the primary indication in 64% (42/66), with rheumatoid arthritis the second most common, accounting for 24% (16/66). The Rebalance Total Ankle Replacement (Zimmer Biomet, Warsaw, IN) was the most commonly used prosthesis, followed by the Trabecular Metal implant (Zimmer Biomet) and the Hintegra prosthesis (Hintegra Total Ankle Replacment, Newdeal, Lyon, France/Integra, Plainsboro, New Jersey), second and third, respectively.

The Swedish Ankle Registry was formalized in 1997 but contains data since 1993. The latest registry report[16] showed a total of 1296 ankle replacements since 1993. During the same time period, 277 (21%) had been revised. However, early data in the registry reflected first-generation, cemented Scandinavian Total Ankle Replacement (STAR; Stryker, Mahwah, NJ) arthroplasties and constrained prostheses that

were subsequently abandoned in the mid-1990s because of poor results. Of the revision cases, 131 (59%) were for prosthesis loosening, 29 (13%) for polyethene wear/fracture, 23 (10%) revised for infection, and 23 (10%) revised for technical failure. Regardless of prosthesis used, overall survival at 5 years was estimated to be 0.81 (81%; 95% confidence interval [CI], 0.79–0.83) and at 10 years 0.69 (69%; 95% CI, 0.67–0.71).

More recently, data have been collected on patient-reported outcome measures (PROMS). Both the foot- and ankle-specific self-reported foot and ankle score (SEFAS) score and EQ-5D score data were published. The SEFAS score raised from a preoperative mean of 16 to a 2-year postoperative score of 31, whereas the EQ-5D score raised from 0.40 to 0.68. Both of these were found to be clinically and statistically significant. PROMS results after revision surgery following a primary replacement were significantly lower.

Two studies analyzing the results after ankle replacement have been published based on data from the Swedish Registry.[17,18] Henricson and colleagues[17] showed a 5-year survival rate of 78% in 531 primary ankle replacements between 1993 and 2005. A long learning curve was demonstrated in that the 5-year prosthetic survival regarding the procedures performed by three surgeons was 70% for their first 30 cases compared with 86% for those performed thereafter. The risk of revision was higher in younger patients than older.[17]

In 2011, Henricson and colleagues[18] showed that the 10-year survival of 780 ankles was estimated to 69%. Excluding the STAR prosthesis (no longer used in Sweden) the 10-year survival was estimated to 78%.[18] It was also demonstrated that women with osteoarthritis and younger than age 60 had a higher risk of revision.[18]

The Norwegian Arthroplasty Register
The Norwegian Joint Registry's latest report was published in 2018.[19] Between 1994 and 2017, 1608 ankle replacements were performed of which 1195 (74.3%) were primary procedures and 413 (25.7%) were revision replacements. Mean age was 59.9 years and 53.9% of procedures were performed in women. In 2017, 50 primary total ankle replacement and 46 revision ankle replacements were performed.

Post-traumatic osteoarthritis was the primary indication accounting for 381 (32%) primary replacements. Idiopathic osteoarthritis accounted for 329 (28%) and rheumatoid arthritis accounted for 321 (27%) replacements. A total of 142 (12%) of the primary replacements were done for the sequalae of ligamentous tear.

Most replacements (1148; 96.1%) were uncemented prostheses. Overall, the most common prosthesis was the Link STAR followed by the Salto Talaris (Integra Lifesciences, Plainsboro, NJ) and the Mobility (Depuy, Raynham, MA) prostheses. More recently (since 2014) the Salto Talaris and the Trabecular Metal Total Ankle were more frequently used.

The most common causes for revision of a primary prosthesis was a proximal (tibial) component (26%; 109/413), a loose distal (talar) component (20%; 83/413), malalignment (16%; 66/413), instability (9.7%; 40/413), and deep infection (8%; 33/413). PROMS data and survivorship data were not published.

The New Zealand Joint Registry
The New Zealand joint registry yearly report published in 2018 included analysis of data from January 2000 to December 2017.[20] During this time, there were a total of 1502 primary ankle arthroplasties registered. The average age for a primary ankle replacement was 66 years (range, 32–96 years), with 39.21% (589 cases) performed in women and 60.79% (913 cases) performed in men. Between 2010 and 2017, 543 primary arthroplasty cases included a documented body mass index, which was found to average 28.44 (17–54).

Osteoarthritis was the most common primary diagnosis found in 1135 (65%) cases with posttrauma being a diagnosis in 240 (16%) and rheumatoid arthritis a diagnosis in a further 126 (8%) cases. Most cases were uncemented with only 25 cemented tibial component and 19 cemented talar components.

In 2017, 122 primary ankle replacement procedures were performed by 20 surgeons. The most commonly used prosthesis was the Salto (Tournier SA, Saint-Ismier, France) followed by the Infinity (Wright Medical Technologies, Memphis, TN).

A total of 167 revisions of primary total ankle procedures were performed during the 18-year period from January 2000 to December 2017. This accounted for around 11% (167/1502). Of the revisions, 42% (70/167) presented with pain, 30% (50/167) had talar component loosening, 22% (36/167) tibial component loosening, and 10% (70/167) and 2% (3/167) had a fracture of the talus.

These registry data suggested a 5- and 10-year overall survivorship of 90.4% and 82.8%, respectively.

The registry previously used a nonvalidated PROMS that was replaced by the Manchester-Oxford Foot Questionnaire toward the end of 2015. As such there were no significant PROMS data available.

The Australian National Joint Replacement Registry
The latest Australian joint registry data were published in a 2018 report[21] of 2474 ankle replacement procedures up to December 31, 2017. This figure included 2014 primary total ankle replacements and 434 revision replacements. Primary total ankle replacement was most commonly performed in men with 1490 (60.2%) of the primary group. The mean age for primary replacement was 67 years (20–94 years).

Overall the most common indication for primary replacement was osteoarthritis (92.9%) with rheumatoid arthritis in second (5.4%). In 2017, 189 primary ankle replacements were performed, with the Salto Talaris (Integra Lifesciences) being the most popular prosthesis, followed by the Hintegra and the Trabecular Metal.

For osteoarthritis, the cumulative percent revision at 5 years was 10.4% and for rheumatoid arthritis was 6.5%. Loosening was the most common cause for revision primary ankle replacements. This accounted for 27.7% of all revisions. Following this, lysis accounted for 10.5% and instability accounted for 9.9% of revisions. Infection took up the fourth most common cause of revision, occurring in 8.9%.

National Joint Registry for England, Wales, Northern Ireland, and the Isle of Man
The latest data available from the UK National joint registry were presented in the 15th annual report published in 2018.[22] This included surgical data up to December 31, 2017. This registry constituted the largest collection of primary ankle arthroplasty of all the registers. In December 2017, there were 4687 primary operations recorded. These were performed by 224 consultant surgeons at 247 orthopedic units. Overall the median age at primary surgery was 68 years (17–93 years). The procedure was more commonly performed in men (59%), and 98.2% of the primary procedures were uncemented.

In 2017, 734 primary operations were performed, an increase on the previous year by 15 cases. The most commonly performed prosthesis during this time was the Infinity (51%), followed by the MatOrtho Box (MatOrtho (Leatherhead, UK) (14.4%) and the STAR Replacement (12.4%).

Table 1
Summary of data from 5 national joint registries for total ankle replacement

Registry	Duration	Total Cases	Latest Year Total Primary Cases	Average Age	Gender	Most Common Indications	Most Common Prostheses in Latest Year	Overall Survivorship
Swedish	1993–2017	1296	66	—	—	OA RA	Rebalance Trabecular Metal Hintegra	81% survival 5 y 69% survival 10 y
Norwegian	1994–2017	1608	50	59.9	53.9% F 46.1% M	Post-traumatic OA Idiopathic OA RA	Salto Talaris Trabecular Metal	
New Zealand	2000–2017	1502	122	66	39.2% F 60.8% M	OA Post-traumatic OA RA	Salto Infinity	90.4% survival 5 y 82.8% survival 10 y
Australia	2006–2017	2474	189	67		OA RA	Salto Talaris Hintegra Trabecular Metal	Revision rate at 5 y 10.4% for OA, 6.5% RA
United Kingdom	2010–2017	4687	734	68	41% F 59% M		Infinity Box STAR	Percentage probability of first revision 6.93 at 5 y 8.70 at 7 y

Abbreviations: OS, osteoarthritis; RA, rheumatoid arthritis.

Of the 4687 primary procedures, only 211 (4.5%) had a linkable national joint registry record to indicate revision of a primary prosthesis. The report noted that the smaller than expected number was likely related to the failure of accurate recording of revision procedures.

The overall estimate of cumulative percentage probability of first revision was found to be 6.93 (95% CI, 6.0–8.0) at 5 years, increasing to 8.70 (95% CI, 7.41–12.0) at 7 years. First revision was found to be more likely in individuals younger than age 65.

Meta-Analyses and Systematic Reviews

As an abstract published in 2018 following an American Orthopedic Foot and Ankle Society (AOFAS) meeting presentation, Gross and colleagues[23] performed a systematic review of the literature addressing the intermediate- to long-term outcomes of interest in total ankle arthroplasty studies published since 2006, and compared findings with earlier generation implants.

The meta-analysis included 40 studies, with a total of 4835 total ankle replacements. The 5- and 10-year survival rates were 86% (P = .001) and 76% (P = .53), respectively. Revision rate was found to be 9.6% (P = .10), more than a third of which were caused by component loosening.

They summarized that the outcomes for third-generation total ankle arthroplasty had no significant differences in survival rates when compared with second-generation implants. However, functional scores, range of motion, and overall patient outcomes were significantly higher in the third-generation implants. To clarify, most second-generation implants were two-component, fixed-bearing systems with a polyethylene bearing surface incorporated into the talar or tibial component, with a preference for press fit designs. Third-generation prostheses were characterized by the addition of a third component, a polyethylene, mobile-bearing meniscus, with more significance placed on ligaments to retain stability.

In 2013, Goldberg and colleagues[24,25] published the results of a meta-analysis of total ankle replacement to determine the survivorship, outcome, complications, radiologic findings, and range of motion in patients with end-stage osteoarthritis undergoing total ankle replacement. A total of 58 studies including 7942 total ankle replacement were reviewed. The mean age at operation was 60 years, with a range from 17 to 95 years.

The most common indication for surgery was found to be post-traumatic osteoarthritis (46%), followed by primary osteoarthritis (27%) and rheumatoid arthritis (19%). The overall 10-year survivorship was found to be 89%.[24] There was an annual failure rate of 1.2% (95% CI, 0.7–1.6). The mean AOFAS score improved from 40 preoperatively to 80 postoperatively, at a mean follow-up of 8 years. This was found to be a statistically significant improvement (P<.01). They also identified a statistically significant improvement in mean total range of ankle joint movement postoperatively. Radiologically, the paper noted a prevalence of lucencies in up to 23% at a mean of 4.4 years. The significance of this finding was unclear. Acknowledging the lack of high-quality randomized controlled trials, the authors commented that total ankle replacement had a positive impact on patient lives with benefits lasting 10 years including improvement in pain and function, and gait.

IMPLANT-SPECIFIC OUTCOMES
Scandinavian Total Ankle Replacement

The STAR has one of the longest histories in total ankle replacement. The most recently published outcome data were published by Clough and colleagues,[26] who reported the long-term clinical and radiologic outcomes of 200 STAR implants from a single center. A total of 184 patients were identified between 1993 and 2000, with prospectively collected data. Eighty-four patients (87 ankles) were contactable by the end of the study. Among these, 16% of implants required revision surgery. Mean time to revision was 80 months and 15.8-year survivorship was 76.16%, with revision surgery as the end point. Mean preoperative AOFAS scores improved from 28 to 61.

Palanca and colleagues[27] identified 84 STAR implants performed between 1998 and 2000. Only 21% (24/84) of these patients achieved the minimum follow-up of 15 years. Fifteen-year survivorship was found to be 73%. AOFAS scores improved from an average of 39.6 points preoperatively, to an average of 71.6 postoperatively. More than half (52.4%) of patients with retained implants required an additional surgical procedure.

Daniels and colleagues[28] prospectively studied consecutive STAR patients between 2001 and 2005. Eleven patients underwent the procedure, with a mean age of 61.9 years. The mean duration of follow-up for all living patients without revision (73 ankles) was 9 years. Thirteen (12%) of the ankles required metal component revision at a mean of 4.3 years. Twenty (18%)

of the prostheses underwent polyethylene bearing exchange, mostly because of fracture, at a mean of 5.2 years.

Hintegra

The Hintegra is a three-component, nonconstrained prosthesis. The polyethylene mobile-bearing provides axial rotation and physiologic flexion and extension mobility, but it also provides inversion and eversion stability.[29] There is no intramedullary fixation of its tibial component, but rather a flat, anatomically shaped component.

In 2013, Barg and colleagues[29] presented overall survival rates of 94% at 5 years and 84 years at 10 years based on a study of 722 Hintegra arthroplasties. There were no polyethylene failures and overall revision rate was 8.4% (61/722). This included three generations of prosthesis and found older generations were at increased risk of earlier revision.

Lefrancois and colleagues[30] published on the outcomes comparing the Agility, Mobility, STAR, and Hintegra. Of 209 Hintegra prostheses the 5-year survival rate was 88%. This is from a nondesigning institution.

Agility Total Ankle Replacement

In 2017, Raikin and colleagues[31] published midterm results of the Agility Total Ankle Replacement. A total of 127 consecutive Agility ankles were included between 2002 and 2009. Ninety (78.2%) of 115 patients retained their primary implant, of which 105 were available for evaluation, with an average follow-up of 9.1 years. An earlier systematic review by Roukis[32] assessed 14 studies with 2312 Agility ankles with a mean follow-up of 22 months. Of the 2312 ankles, 224 (9.7%) underwent revision. When inventor and noninventor studies were separated, the revision rate doubled from 6.6% to 12.2%, respectively.

The study by Lefrancois and colleagues[30] on the outcomes comparing the Agility, Mobility, STAR, and Hintegra found that of 63 Agility prostheses the 5-year survival rate was 88%, and 10 years was 79%.

Salto/Salto Talaris

The mobile-bearing Salto and its fixed-bearing variant the Salto Talaris are current third-generation implants in common use. A systematic review performed to assess the incidence of revision after implantation of both systems identified eight studies with 1209 Saltos and five studies with 212 Salto Talaris implants, with weighted mean follow-ups of 55.2 and

34.9 months, respectively.[33] Forty-eight (4%) of the Salto and five (2.4%) of the Salto Talaris implants required revision. When data were subdivided into inventor/disclosed consultant and nondesign team, there was a lower revision rate in the nondesign team group, suggesting the absence of inventor bias.

Stewart and colleagues[34] published in 2017 on midterm results of the Salto Talaris. They identified 72 patients, with a mean age of 61.9 years and mean follow-up of 81.1 months. Survivorship was 95.8% for those with at least 5-year follow-up, with two patients undergoing revision arthroplasty for aseptic loosening and a third patient scheduled for revision for a chronic wound infection. Fourteen patients (19%) required an additional surgery for a total of 17 additional operative procedures on the ipsilateral ankle or hindfoot. Hofmann and colleagues[35] published a retrospective analysis of 81 Salto Talaris ankles with a minimum 2-year follow-up. Implant survival was 97.5% at a mean follow-up time of 5.2 years. There was one revision of a tibial component and one revision of a talar component. Thirty-six (44.4%) patients underwent additional procedures at time of joint replacement, most commonly removal of hardware. Seventeen (20.9%) patients underwent further surgery, most commonly gutter debridement.

In 2018, Wan and colleagues[36] published their results on the mobile-bearing Salto. The retrospective study on 59 Salto implants with a mean follow-up of 35.9 months showed promising early clinical results. By the last follow-up, 7 of 59 patients (11.9%) had undergone reoperation, and 3 of 59 implants (5.1%) had been removed. The prosthesis survival was 94.9% (95% CI, 89.1%–100%). With any reoperation as the end point of follow-up, the clinical success rate was 88.1% (95% CI, 79.4%–96.9%). The mean postoperative Visual Analog Scale score, AOFAS ankle-hindfoot score, and Ankle Osteoarthritis Scale pain and disability score improved significantly ($P<.001$). The ankle range of motion also improved from preoperative; however, there was no statistically significant change in plantarflexion.

Another study from the same year by Koo and colleagues[37] reported on 50 consecutive patients with 55 Salto implants and a minimum 5-year follow-up. Six implants were lost to follow-up. Three (6.1%) implants were revised for aseptic loosening (in two cases) or infection. Two (4%) further patients underwent reoperations, one for arthroscopic debridement of anterolateral synovitis and one for grafting of an asymptomatic tibial cyst. With all-cause revision as an end point, implant survival was 93.3% at 5 to 10 years (95% CI, 80.5%–97.8%). When reoperations were included this fell to 90.2% (95% CI, 75.6%–96.3%) at 5 years.

Infinity Total Ankle Replacement

The Infinity total ankle replacement is a newer fixed-bearing prosthesis. The first clinical results were published in 2018 by Penner and colleagues[38] who presented early clinical results from 67 patients between 2013 and 2015. The overall implant survival rate was 97% (65 of 67 implants) at a mean follow-up of 35.4 months (27–47 months). Two cases underwent talar component revision for aseptic loosening. Six of the 67 cases (9%) required a nonrevision reoperation. A subsequent paper by Saito and colleagues[39] retrospectively reviewed 64 consecutive primary Infinity total ankle arthroplasty from July 2014 to April 2016. Average follow-up was 24.5 months, although minimum follow-up was only 18 months. Survivorship of the implant was 95.3%. Fourteen ankles (21.8%) presented a total of 17 complications. A total of 12 reoperations were necessary in 11 ankles (17.1%). Revision surgery was indicated for three ankles (4.7%) as a result of subsidence of the implant. Outcome scores were significantly improved for all Foot & Ankle Outcome Score components. On closer review, these improved from 39.0 to 83.3 for pain, from 34.0 to 65.2 for symptoms, from 52.3 to 87.5 for activities of daily living, and from 15.7 to 64.2 for quality of life.

Cody and colleagues[40] reported a series of 159 Infinity total ankle replacements with only a minimum of 12 month follow-up with only 6 of 159 cases (3.8%) revised for loosening. However, their results showed a high rate of revision for deep infection (3.8%) and showed revision surgery for other causes as early as 5 months postoperative. In view of these findings, and the reported rate of nearly one-third of the failed cases being implanted incorrectly (ie, left in approximately 5° of varus tilt, reportedly shown on 6-week postoperative radiographs), the reliability of this report has been questioned.[41]

Trabecular Metal

In addition to the previously mentioned established prosthesis, there are several newer prosthesis that are gaining popularity. Barg and colleagues[42] present a therapeutic level-IV cohort analysis of the short-term clinical and radiographic outcomes of 54 patients (55 ankles) undergoing TAA with use of a novel transfibular surgical approach, with a mean follow-up of 26.6 months. This was using the Trabecular Metal (Zimmer Biomet) implant, which as the name suggests is a prosthesis made of trabecular metal. The two innovative aspects here are the transfibular approach and the trabecular metal prosthesis to encourage bony ingrowth.

Implant survival was 93% at 2 years. Three implants (5.5%) were revised for aseptic loosing, because of lack of bony ingrowth. In 10 of the 55 cases (18%), a secondary procedure was performed during follow-up. No delayed union or nonunion was observed for fibular healing. Overall complication rate was 11%. The average Visual Analog Scale pain score decreased significantly, as did the average total range of motion of the ankle.

Usuelli and colleagues[43] published in 2019 on 89 Trabecular Metal replacements at average follow-up of 42 months. A 98.9% of patients were free of component removal or revision at final follow-up, with one revision for infection, and no revisions for aseptic loosening.

DISCUSSION

Modern-generation ankle replacements have seemingly encouraging results based on registry data and the general literature. As the failings of the first-generation implants have been improved on, there have been better outcomes and survival rates. However, the available pool of data presents several issues.

National joint registry data on total ankle replacements provides important information and surveillance on the outcomes of total ankle arthroplasty. It must be recognized, however, that these data have limitations. There is debate on how accurately the data reflect current practice, lack of PROMs, and the incomplete capture of the true picture, with somewhat hard end points. A report by Muir in 2017[44] identified several issues with registry data for ankle replacements, including data confounders and data capture problems especially with underreporting of revision procedures.

Despite the advances made in total ankle arthroplasty design and implantation, the previous poor results from earlier generations of prosthesis will have a negative effect on overall survival and revision rates. As pointed out by Zaidi and colleagues,[23] registries include a wide range of data from surgeons, including those carrying out small volumes, and surgeons who are within their learning curves and would be expected to have higher rates of failure.

The incomplete capture of revision procedures also somewhat muddies the picture.

Unfortunately, the wider literature does not provide a significantly more accurate data source. Most studies are level IV evidence of largely case series, and there is an absence of prospective, randomized-controlled, level I data.

There is only one large, nonindustry sponsored prospective mid- to long-term study of total ankle replacement outcomes compared with ankle arthrodesis, the only current alternative to total ankle replacement.[45] These results, although not stratified, show even second-generation total ankle replacement implants to have outcomes at least as good as arthrodesis. Further data have been presented to suggest that with third-generation implants, patient-reported outcomes for total ankle replacement may be superior to arthrodesis with both having similar mid-term revision rates.[46]

Heterogeneity of outcome measures makes direct comparison of outcomes challenging. Whether revision is defined as reoperation rather than more specifically removal of implants affects prosthesis survival rates. Inventor/design team data and conversely competing design team data may introduce inherent bias.

Current evidence does not support the use of one prosthesis over another, nor one group of prostheses over another. Total ankle replacement as a treatment of ankle arthritis is a safe and reliable technique, with encouraging outcomes. As has been the case for some time, further high-quality studies are required to clarify outcomes post ankle arthroplasty. Stratification of outcomes by ankle deformity or varying degrees of ankle arthritis complexity, as defined by the COFAS Ankle Arthritis Classification,[46] or for patients with comorbidities, such as diabetes, obesity, and peripheral vascular disease, may help to identify those who will likely have better outcomes or be predisposed to implant failure or other adverse events.

DISCLOSURES

None (L. Jeyaseelan, S. Si-Hyeong Park, H. Al-Rumaih). Arthrex, Inc: paid presenter or speaker. Arthritis Innovation Corporation: stock or stock options, Therapia: stock or stock options (A. Veljkovic). Amniox: paid consultant; paid presenter or speaker; research support. Arthrex, Inc: other financial or material support. Canadian Orthopedic Foot & Ankle Society: board or committee member. Cartiva: other financial or material support. International Federation of Foot & Ankle Societies: board or committee member. Springer: publishing royalties, financial or material support. Synthes: other financial or material support. Wright Medical Technology, Inc: IP royalties; paid consultant; paid presenter or speaker; research support. Zimmer: other financial or material support (M.J. Penner). Wright Medical: consultant. Arthrex, Acumed, Johnson & Johnson: research office support (K.J. Wing). Acumed, LLC: paid consultant; paid presenter or speaker; research support. American Orthopedic Foot and Ankle Society: board or committee member. Amniox: research support. Bioventus: paid consultant; research support. Canadian Orthopedic Association: board or committee member. Cartiva: research support. CONMED Linvatec: paid presenter or speaker. Ferring Pharmaceuticals: paid consultant; paid presenter or speaker; research support. Foot and Ankle International: editorial or governing board. Stryker: paid presenter or speaker. Synthes: research support. Wolters Kluwer Health - Lippincott Williams & Wilkins: editorial or governing board. Wright Medical Technology, Inc: paid consultant; paid presenter or speaker; research support. Zimmer: paid consultant; paid presenter or speaker; research support (A. Younger).

REFERENCES

1. Saltzman CL, Zimmerman MB, O'Rourke M, et al. Impact of comorbidities on the measurement of health in patients with ankle osteoarthritis. J Bone Joint Surg Am 2006;88-11:2366–72.

2. Glazebrook M, Daniels T, Younger A, et al. Comparison of health-related quality of life between patients with end-stage ankle and hip arthrosis. J Bone Joint Surg Am 2008;90(3):499–505.

3. Goldberg AJ, Macgregor A, Dawson J, et al. The demand incidence of symptomatic ankle osteoarthritis presenting to foot & ankle surgeons in the United Kingdom. Foot (Edinb) 2012;22-3:163–6.

4. Barg A, Pagenstert GI, Hügle T, et al. Ankle osteoarthritis: etiology, diagnostics, and classification. Foot Ankle Clin 2013;18:411–26.

5. Saltzman CL, Salamon ML, Blanchard GM, et al. Epidemiology of ankle arthritis: report of a consecutive series of 639 patients from a tertiary orthopaedic center. Iowa Orthop J 2005;25:44–6.

6. Harrington KD. Degenerative arthritis of the ankle secondary to long-standing lateral ligament instability. J Bone Joint Surg Am 1979;61(3):354–61.

7. Valderrabano V, Hintermann B, Horisberger M, et al. Ligamentous posttraumatic ankle osteoarthritis. Am J Sports Med 2006;34(4):612–20.

8. Fuchs S, Sandmann CM, Skwara A, et al. Quality of life 20 years after arthrodesis of the ankle. A study

of adjacent joints. J Bone Joint Surg Br 2003;85(7): 994–8.

9. Hendrickx RP, Stufkens SA, de Bruijn EE. Medium to long-term outcome of ankle arthrodesis. Foot Ankle Int 2011;32(10):940–7.

10. Barg A, Wimmer MD, Wiewiorski M, et al. Total ankle replacement: indications, implant designs, and results. Dtsch Arztebl Int 2015;112:177.

11. Hopgood P, Kumar R, Wood P. Ankle arthrodesis for failed total ankle replacement. J Bone Joint Surg Br 2006;88:1032–8.

12. Helm R, Stevens J. Long-term results of total ankle replacement. J Arthroplasty 1986;1:271–7.

13. Kotnis R, Pasapula C, Anwar F, et al. The management of failed ankle replacement. J Bone Joint Surg Br 2006;88:1039–47.

14. Courville XF, Hecht PJ, Tosteson AN. Is total ankle arthroplasty a cost-effective alternative to ankle fusion? Clin Orthop Relat Res 2011;469:1721–7.

15. Saltzman CL, Kadoko RG, Suh JS. Treatment of isolated ankle osteoarthritis with arthrodesis or the total ankle replacement: a comparison of early outcomes. Clin Orthop Relat Res 2010;2:1–7.

16. SwedAnkle. The Swedish Ankle Registry Annual Report 2017. Available at: http://www.swedankle.se. Accessed May 2019.

17. Henricson A, Skoog A, Carlsson Å. The Swedish Ankle Arthroplasty Register. An analysis of 531 arthroplasties between 1993 and 2005. Acta Orthop 2007;78:569–74.

18. Henricson A, Nilsson J-Å, Carlsson Å. 10-year survival of total ankle arthroplasties. A report on 780 cases from the Swedish Ankle Register. Acta Orthop 2011;82:655–9.

19. Norwegian National Advisory Unit on Arthroplasty and Hip Fractures Report 2018. Available at: http://nrlweb.ihelse.net/eng/. Accessed May 2019.

20. The New Zealand Joint Registry. 19th Year Report, January 1999 to December 2017. Available at: https://nzoa.org.nz/nzoa-joint-registry. Accessed May 2019.

21. National Joint Replacement Registry. Demographics and outcomes of ankle arthroplasty: supplementary report 2018. Australian Orthopaedic Association. Available at: https://aoanjrr.sahmri.com/annual-reports-2018/supplementary. Accessed May 2019.

22. National joint registry for England, Wales, Northern Ireland and the Isle of Man. 15th annual report 2018. Surgical data to 31 December 2017. Available at: www.njrcentre.org.uk. Accessed May 2019.

23. Zaidi R, Cro S, Gurusamy K, et al. The outcome of total ankle replacement: a systematic review and meta-analysis. Bone Joint J 2013;95-B(11): 1500–7.

24. Gross C, Haddad S, Morris J, et al. A 27-year Meta-analysis of Ankle Arthroplasty. Foot & Ankle Orthopaedics 2018;3(3).

25. Gittins J, Mann RA. The history of the STAR total ankle arthroplasty. Foot Ankle Clin 2002;7:809–16.

26. Clough T, Bodo K, Majeed H, et al. Survivorship and long-term outcome of a consecutive series of 200 Scandinavian Total Ankle Replacement (STAR) implants. Bone Joint J 2019;101-B(1):47–54.

27. Palanca A, Mann RA, Mann JA, et al. Scandinavian total ankle replacement: 15-year follow-up. Foot Ankle Int 2018;39(2):135–42.

28. Daniels TR, Mayich DJ, Penner MJ. Intermediate to long-term outcomes of total ankle replacement with the Scandinavian Total Ankle Replacement (STAR). J Bone Joint Surg Am 2015;97(11):895–903.

29. Barg A, Zwicky L, Knupp M, et al. HINTEGRA total ankle replacement: survivorship analysis in 684 patients. J Bone Joint Surg Am 2013;95(13):1175–83.

30. Lefrancois T, Younger A, Wing K, et al. A prospective study of four total ankle arthroplasty implants by non-designer investigators. J Bone Joint Surg Am 2017;99(4):342–8.

31. Raikin SM, Sandrowski K, Kane JM, et al. Midterm outcome of the Agility total ankle arthroplasty. Foot Ankle Int 2017;38(6):662–70.

32. Roukis TS. Incidence of revision after primary implantation of the Agility total ankle replacement system: a systematic review. J Foot Ankle Surg 2012;51(2):198–204.

33. Roukis TS, Elliott AD. Incidence of revision after primary implantation of the Salto Mobile Version and Salto Talaris total ankle prostheses: a systematic review. J Foot Ankle Surg 2015;54(3):311–9.

34. Stewart MG, Green CL, Adams SB, et al. Midterm results of the Salto Talaris total ankle arthroplasty. Foot Ankle Int 2017;38(11):1215–21.

35. Hofmann KJ, Shabin ZM, Ferkel E, et al. Salto Talaris total ankle arthroplasty: clinical results at a mean of 5.2 years in 78 patients treated by a single surgeon. J Bone Joint Surg Am 2016; 98(24):2036–46.

36. Wan DD, Choi WJ, Shim DW, et al. Short-term clinical and radiographic results of the Salto mobile total ankle prosthesis. Foot Ankle Int 2017;39(2):155–65.

37. Koo K, Liddle AD, Pastides PS, et al. The Salto total ankle arthroplasty: clinical and radiological outcomes at five years. Foot Ankle Surg 2018. [Epub ahead of print].

38. Penner M, Davis WH, Wing K, et al. The Infinity total ankle system: early clinical results with 2- to 4-year follow-up. Foot Ankle Spec 2019;12(2):159–66.

39. King A, Bali N, Kassam AA, et al. Early outcomes and radiographic alignment of the Infinity total ankle replacement with a minimum of two year follow-up data. Foot Ankle Surg 2018 [pii:S1268-7731(18)30082-1].

40. Cody EA, Taylor MA, Nunley JA 2nd, et al. Increased early revision rate with the INFINITY total ankle prosthesis. Foot Ankle Int 2019;40(1):9–17.

41. Haddad SL. Letter regarding: increased early revision rate with the INFINITY total ankle prosthesis. Foot Ankle Int 2019;40(1):124–6.

42. Barg A, Bettin CC, Burstein AH, et al. Early clinical and radiographic outcomes of trabecular metal total ankle replacement using a transfibular approach. J Bone Joint Surg Am 2018;100(6): 505–15.

43. Usuelli FG, Maccario C, Granata F, et al. Clinical and radiological outcomes of transfibular total ankle arthroplasty. Foot Ankle Int 2019;40(1):24–33.

44. Muir D. Is there anything to learn from a national joint registry? Foot Ankle Clin 2017;22(2):465–75.

45. Daniels TR, Younger AS, Penner M, et al. Intermediate-term results of total ankle replacement and ankle arthrodesis: a COFAS multicenter study. J Bone Joint Surg Am 2014;96(2):135–42.

46. Krause FG, Di Silvestro M, Penner M, et al. Inter- and intraobserver reliability of the COFAS end-stage ankle arthritis classification system. Foot Ankle Int 2010;31(2):103–8. AOFAS Meeting Abstracts 2018.

UNITED STATES POSTAL SERVICE ® Statement of Ownership, Management, and Circulation (All Periodicals Publications Except Requester Publications)

1. Publication Title	2. Publication Number		3. Filing Date
ORTHOPEDIC CLINICS OF NORTH AMERICA	950 – 920		9/18/2019

4. Issue Frequency	5. Number of Issues Published Annually	6. Annual Subscription Price
JAN, APR, JUL, OCT	4	$341.00

7. Complete Mailing Address of Known Office of Publication (Not printer) (Street, city, county, state, and ZIP+4®)

ELSEVIER INC.
230 Park Avenue, Suite 800
New York, NY 10169

Contact Person
STEPHEN R. BUSHING

Telephone (Include area code)
215-239-3688

8. Complete Mailing Address of Headquarters or General Business Office of Publisher (Not printer)

ELSEVIER INC.
230 Park Avenue, Suite 800
New York, NY 10169

9. Full Names and Complete Mailing Addresses of Publisher, Editor, and Managing Editor (Do not leave blank)

Publisher (Name and complete mailing address)

TAYLOR BALL, ELSEVIER INC.
1600 JOHN F KENNEDY BLVD. SUITE 1800
PHILADELPHIA, PA 19103-2899

Editor (Name and complete mailing address)

LAUREN BOYLE, ELSEVIER INC.
1600 JOHN F KENNEDY BLVD. SUITE 1800
PHILADELPHIA, PA 19103-2899

Managing Editor (Name and complete mailing address)

PATRICK MANLEY, ELSEVIER INC.
1600 JOHN F KENNEDY BLVD. SUITE 1800
PHILADELPHIA, PA 19103-2899

10. Owner (Do not leave blank. If the publication is owned by a corporation, give the name and address of the corporation immediately followed by the names and addresses of all stockholders owning or holding 1 percent or more of the total amount of stock. If not owned by a corporation, give the names and addresses of the individual owners. If owned by a partnership or other unincorporated firm, give its name and address as well as those of each individual owner. If the publication is published by a nonprofit organization, give its name and address.)

Full Name	Complete Mailing Address
WHOLLY OWNED SUBSIDIARY OF REED/ELSEVIER, US HOLDINGS	1600 JOHN F KENNEDY BLVD. SUITE 1800 PHILADELPHIA, PA 19103-2899

11. Known Bondholders, Mortgagees, and Other Security Holders Owning or Holding 1 Percent or More of Total Amount of Bonds, Mortgages, or Other Securities. If none, check box ▶ ☐ None

Full Name	Complete Mailing Address
N/A	

12. Tax Status (For completion by nonprofit organizations authorized to mail at nonprofit rates) (Check one)
The purpose, function, and nonprofit status of this organization and the exempt status for federal income tax purposes:
☒ Has Not Changed During Preceding 12 Months
☐ Has Changed During Preceding 12 Months (Publisher must submit explanation of change with this statement)

PS Form 3526, July 2014 (Page 1 of 4 (see instructions page 4)) PSN: 7530-01-000-9931   PRIVACY NOTICE: See our privacy policy on www.usps.com.

13. Publication Title	14. Issue Date for Circulation Data Below
ORTHOPEDIC CLINICS OF NORTH AMERICA	JULY 2019

15. Extent and Nature of Circulation			Average No. Copies Each Issue During Preceding 12 Months	No. Copies of Single Issue Published Nearest to Filing Date
a. Total Number of Copies (Net press run)			288	245
b. Paid Circulation (By Mail and Outside the Mail)	(1)	Mailed Outside-County Paid Subscriptions Stated on PS Form 3541 (include paid distribution above nominal rate, advertiser's proof copies, and exchange copies)	88	69
	(2)	Mailed In-County Paid Subscriptions Stated on PS Form 3541 (include paid distribution above nominal rate, advertiser's proof copies, and exchange copies)	0	0
	(3)	Paid Distribution Outside the Mails Including Sales Through Dealers and Carriers, Street Vendors, Counter Sales, and Other Paid Distribution Outside USPS®	119	125
	(4)	Paid Distribution by Other Classes of Mail Through the USPS (e.g., First-Class Mail®)	0	0
c. Total Paid Distribution (Sum of 15b (1), (2), (3), and (4))		▶	207	194
d. Free or Nominal Rate Distribution (By Mail and Outside the Mail)	(1)	Free or Nominal Rate Outside-County Copies included on PS Form 3541	68	33
	(2)	Free or Nominal Rate In-County Copies Included on PS Form 3541	0	0
	(3)	Free or Nominal Rate Copies Mailed at Other Classes Through the USPS (e.g., First-Class Mail)	0	0
	(4)	Free or Nominal Rate Distribution Outside the Mail (Carriers or other means)	0	0
e. Total Free or Nominal Rate Distribution (Sum of 15d (1), (2), (3) and (4))		▶	68	33
f. Total Distribution (Sum of 15c and 15e)		▶	275	227
g. Copies not Distributed (See instructions to Publishers #4 (page #3))		▶	13	18
h. Total (Sum of 15f and g)		▶	288	245
i. Percent Paid (15c divided by 15f times 100)		▶	75.27%	85.46%

* If you are claiming electronic copies, go to line 16 on page 3. If you are not claiming electronic copies, skip to line 17 on page 3.

16. Electronic Copy Circulation	Average No. Copies Each Issue During Preceding 12 Months	No. Copies of Single Issue Published Nearest to Filing Date
a. Paid Electronic Copies ▶		
b. Total Paid Print Copies (Line 15c) + Paid Electronic Copies (Line 16a) ▶		
c. Total Print Distribution (Line 15f) + Paid Electronic Copies (Line 16a) ▶		
d. Percent Paid (Both Print & Electronic Copies) (16b divided by 16c × 100) ▶		

☒ I certify that 50% of all my distributed copies (electronic and print) are paid above a nominal price.

17. Publication of Statement of Ownership

☒ If the publication is a general publication, publication of this statement is required. Will be printed in the OCTOBER 2019 issue of this publication.   ☐ Publication not required.

18. Signature and Title of Editor, Publisher, Business Manager, or Owner

STEPHEN R. BUSHING - INVENTORY DISTRIBUTION CONTROL MANAGER

Date 9/18/2019

I certify that all information furnished on this form is true and complete. I understand that anyone who furnishes false or misleading information on this form or who omits material or information requested on the form may be subject to criminal sanctions (including fines and imprisonment) and/or civil sanctions (including civil penalties).

PS Form 3526, July 2014 (Page 3 of 4)   PRIVACY NOTICE: See our privacy policy on www.usps.com.

Moving?

Make sure your subscription moves with you!

To notify us of your new address, find your **Clinics Account Number** (located on your mailing label above your name), and contact customer service at:

Email: journalscustomerservice-usa@elsevier.com

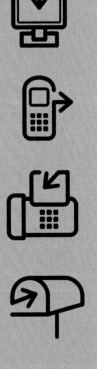

800-654-2452 (subscribers in the U.S. & Canada)
314-447-8871 (subscribers outside of the U.S. & Canada)

Fax number: 314-447-8029

Elsevier Health Sciences Division
Subscription Customer Service
3251 Riverport Lane
Maryland Heights, MO 63043

ELSEVIER

Printed and bound by CPI Group (UK) Ltd, Croydon, CR0 4YY

08/05/2025

01864747-0014